Table of Contents

BLS Care

Additional Considerations

Additional Information

Sudden Cardiac Arrest

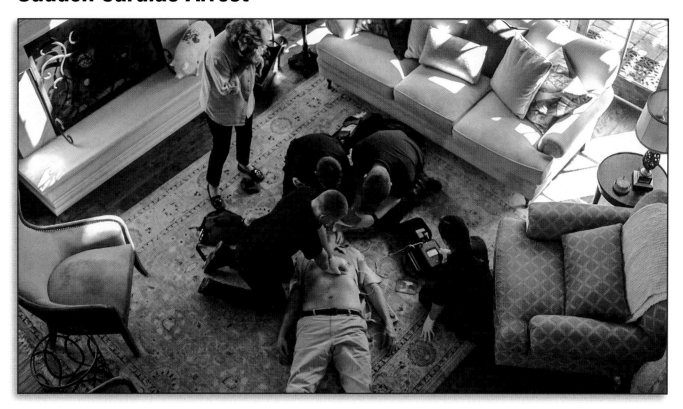

Cardiac arrest is the loss of the heart's ability to pump blood through the body. The most dramatic occurrence, sudden cardiac arrest, can happen anywhere with little or no warning. Victims unexpectedly collapse. Breathing stops.

Sudden cardiac arrest occurs when the normal electrical impulses in the heart suddenly become disorganized. Normal mechanical contraction of the heart muscle is lost, and a chaotic, quivering condition known as ventricular fibrillation can occur. Blood flow to the body, along with the oxygen it carries, abruptly stops. Within minutes, brain cell death starts to occur from the lack of oxygen.

Cardiopulmonary Resuscitation (CPR)

Cardiopulmonary resuscitation (CPR) is the immediate treatment for a suspected cardiac arrest. CPR can restore limited oxygen to the brain and other vital organs through a combination of chest compressions and rescue breaths. However, CPR alone is not enough.

Early Defibrillation

The most effective way to end fibrillation is defibrillation, using a defibrillator and electrode pads adhered to the chest. A controlled electrical shock is sent through the heart to stop ventricular fibrillation, allowing the heart's normal electrical activity to return and restore the normal pumping action of the heart.

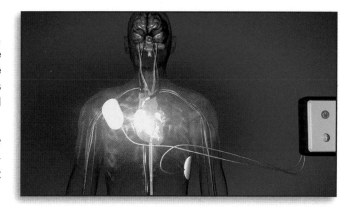

Successful defibrillation is highly dependent on how quickly a shock can be delivered. For each minute in cardiac arrest, the chance of surviving goes down by about 10%. After as few as 10 minutes, survival is unlikely.

An automated external defibrillator (AED) is a portable, computerized device that is simple to operate. The use of AEDs by emergency responders and other healthcare personnel allows defibrillation to occur much earlier than before.

Turning on an AED is as simple as pushing a power button. Once on, an AED provides voice instructions to guide an operator through its use. An AED automatically analyzes the heart rhythm to determine if a shock is needed. If a shock is advised by the AED, the operator clears the person and pushes a button to deliver the shock.

Ventricular Tachycardia

Ventricular tachycardia (VT) occurs when the bottom portion of the heart beats at a very fast rate. In extreme cases, it beats so fast that the heart's ability to actually move blood forward is lost, resulting in cardiac arrest. Just as with ventricular fibrillation, high-quality CPR and early defibrillation are the indicated treatments for VT.

Chain of Survival

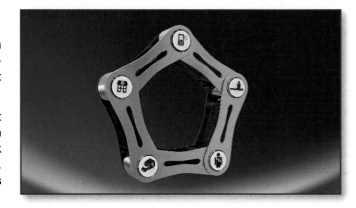

Immediate high-quality CPR and early defibrillation with an AED can double or even triple the likelihood for survival. Most cardiac arrests occur outside of a hospital. Most of those occur in the home.

The chain of survival is often used to describe the best approach for treating cardiac arrest. Each link in the chain is essential for a person to survive. If a single link is weak or missing, the chances for survival are greatly reduced. The greatest chance for survival exists when all the links are strong.

The chain of survival for cardiac arrests outside of a hospital consists of 5 interdependent links:

- Early recognition of cardiac arrest and prompt activation of the emergency response protocol for the setting
- Immediate CPR with high-quality chest compressions
- Rapid defibrillation, or electrical shock, to the heart
- Effective basic and advanced EMS care and transport
- Effective post-cardiac arrest care at a hospital

Cardiac arrest inside a hospital usually occurs when a known medical condition worsens. The chain of survival inside a hospital reflects how resuscitation fits into the overall picture of medical care:

- Monitoring, prevention, and treatment of prearrest conditions
- Early recognition of cardiac arrest and prompt activation of the emergency response protocol for the setting
- Immediate CPR with high-quality chest compressions
- Rapid defibrillation, or electrical shock, to the heart
- Effective post-cardiac arrest care

Knowledge Check

What is the most effective way to end ventricular fibrillation?

Secondary Cardiac Arrest

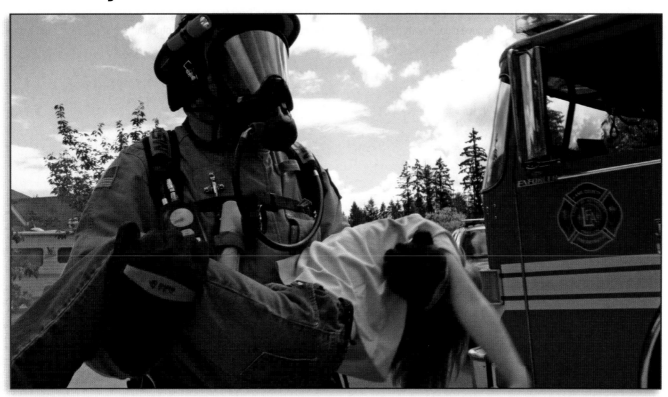

Unlike sudden cardiac arrest in which the heart is the primary problem, cardiac arrest can also be the end result of a blocked airway or loss of breathing. This is known as secondary cardiac arrest.

Problems such as hazardous breathing conditions in a confined space, drowning, and drug overdoses are all causes of secondary cardiac arrest. With no incoming oxygen, the heart progressively becomes weaker until signs of life become difficult or impossible to assess.

If the heart is simply too weak to create obvious signs of life, immediate CPR, with an emphasis on effective rescue breaths, may be the only chance to restore them.

Children and Infants

Children are more likely than adults to experience secondary cardiac arrest due to an airway or breathing problem.

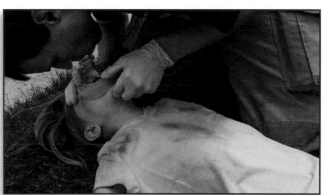

When describing age groups in relation to CPR, an infant is younger than 1 year of age. A child is 1 year of age until the onset of puberty. Puberty can be identified by breast development in females and the presence of armpit hair in males. A person is considered an adult after the onset of puberty.

The chain of survival for children and infants emphasizes prevention and giving effective rescue breaths as part of CPR:

- Prevention of airway and breathing emergencies
- Early CPR, with an emphasis on effective rescue breaths, and, if needed, defibrillation with an AED
- Prompt activation of the emergency response protocol for the setting
- Effective basic and advanced EMS care and transport
- Effective post-cardiac arrest care at a hospital

Opioid Overdose

The abuse of opioid drugs is a serious and growing health problem. Increasing prescriptions for opioid pain relievers, such as hydrocodone and oxycodone, have made them more commonly available. The increased availability and use of heroin, a highly addictive opioid, is also contributing to the problem.

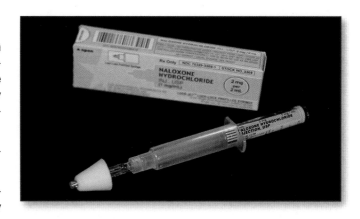

As a result, overdoses and deaths from prescription opioids and heroin have risen dramatically.

Opioids, taken in excess, can depress and stop breathing. Opioid overdose is a common cause of secondary cardiac arrest.

Naloxone, also known as Narcan, is a medication that can temporarily reverse the life-threatening effects of opioids. It is easy to administer, either through an auto-injector device or through an aerosol that is sprayed into the nose.

Suspicion of opioid use may present itself through questioning of bystanders, or by observation of the person and location in which he or she was found. Initiate and establish BLS care prior to using naloxone for a suspected opioid overdose.

Knowledge Check

A 34-year-old man has been pulled out of a lake after being submerged for several minutes. Bystanders describe that he appeared to become exhausted while swimming. Why are effective rescue breaths important if your BLS assessment indicates cardiac arrest?

High-Performance CPR

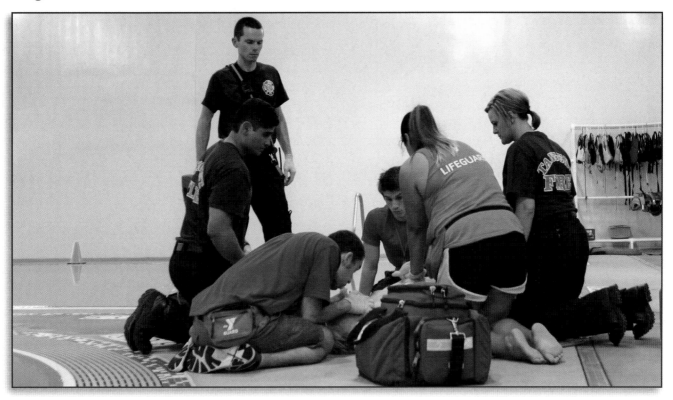

The quality of CPR matters. Higher quality CPR performance is directly related to an improved chance of survival.

There are 2 key elements of high-performance CPR:

- High-quality CPR skills
- A more efficient team approach to resuscitation

High-Quality CPR Skills

CPR skills can vary greatly, depending on a person's experience, practice, and physical ability. It is normal for there to be a gap between perfect skills and what you can actually perform. An important goal is to narrow that gap as much as possible.

High-quality CPR skills include the following:

- Beginning CPR compressions within 10 seconds of determining cardiac arrest
- Compressing fast, at a rate of 100 to 120 times per minute
- Compressing hard, at least 2 inches on an adult, and at least 1/3 the depth of the chest for children and infants
- Allowing for complete chest recoil at the top of each compression
- Minimizing any interruptions to compressions
- Giving effective rescue breaths that create a visible chest rise
- Avoiding excessive air on rescue breaths

CPR feedback devices that measure skill performance in real time can be used to optimize CPR.

Working as a Team

High-quality skills are only part of high-performance CPR. Orchestrating the actions of a resuscitation through a team approach, much like a pit crew in a car race, can significantly improve the care being provided.

An effective team approach

- has clearly defined roles,
- uses clear and effective communication,
- allows multiple treatment actions to occur at the same time,
- maintains high-quality CPR by allowing team members to switch places when tired, and
- minimizes overall interruption times.

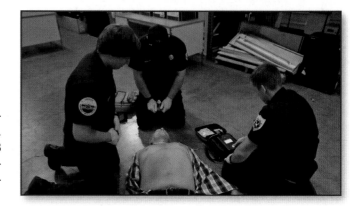

The only way to develop a high-performance CPR approach is through ongoing commitment and practice. CPR skills can deteriorate significantly in as few as 3 months. Shorter, more frequent, scenario-based retraining sessions are reasonable for maintaining skills for individuals likely to respond to a cardiac arrest.

Knowledge Check

You are part of a team of BLS providers who have responded to a person experiencing a cardiac arrest. Identify the 2 main things that have an influence on being able to treat this person in a high-performance manner.

PREPARING TO RESPOND

Protecting Yourself

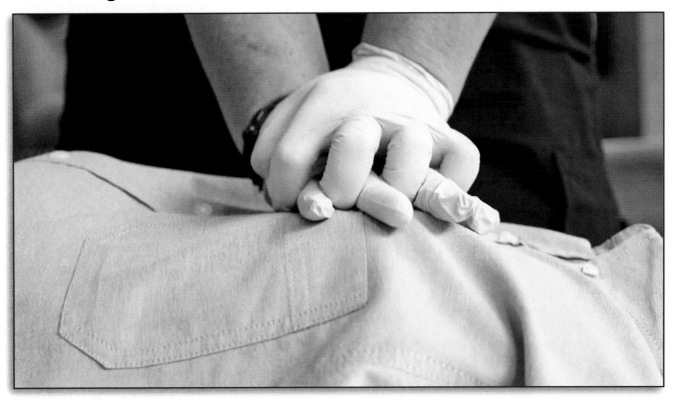

Emergency situations often present hazards to your safety and health. Understanding this and taking simple precautions can significantly reduce your risk.

Personal Safety

Your personal safety is the highest priority, even before the safety of an ill or injured person. Putting yourself in danger to help someone can make the situation worse.

Always pause for a moment before approaching. Look for obvious hazards. Consider the possibility of hidden dangers. If the scene is not safe, do not enter it until hazards have been minimized or eliminated.

Standard Precautions

When caring for someone, you can be exposed to blood or other potentially infectious body fluids. While the risk of contracting a disease is very low, you must take measures to reduce exposure.

The most common infectious bloodborne diseases and pathogens include hepatitis B, hepatitis C, and HIV, the virus that causes AIDS.

Standard precautions are protective practices used when providing care whether or not an infection is suspected.

Personal Protective Equipment (PPE)

Personal protective equipment (PPE) describes protective barriers worn to prevent exposure to infectious diseases. Reducing exposure lowers the chance of infection. Disposable gloves are the most commonly used barrier. Make sure they are readily available and always use them.

Unprotected mouth-to-mouth rescue breaths should not be given by emergency response personnel.[1] Use a CPR mask with a one-way valve when giving rescue breaths or a bag-mask device to prevent direct mouth-to-mouth contact.

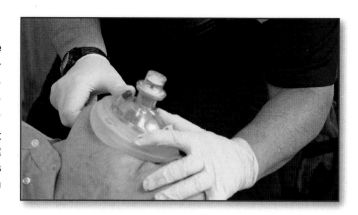

Resuscitation PPE

Common PPE for resuscitation includes disposable gloves, CPR masks, bag-mask devices, protective eyewear, and face shields.

Knowledge Check

True or false? You are caring for a 5-year-old child who is not breathing. Because she is a child it is not important to use a CPR mask or bag-mask device when giving rescue breaths.

PREPARING TO RESPOND

Calling for Help

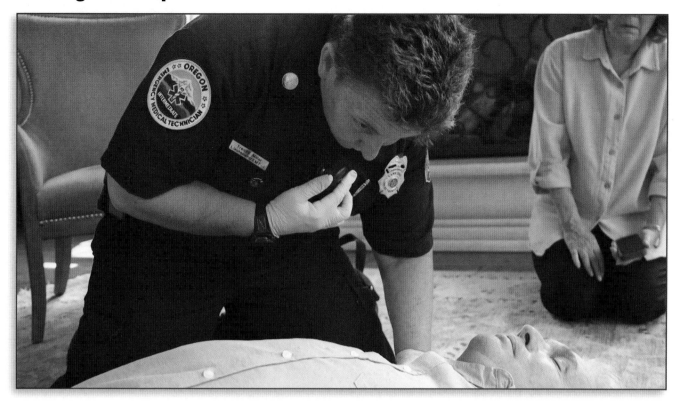

BLS providers, and the locations in which they work, vary. So do the ways in which they activate responses for higher levels of care.

Activation is typically defined by emergency response protocol:

- A BLS provider or member of a workplace emergency response team may radio a centralized communication person to contact EMS, or the provider may call EMS directly.

- An EMS provider may request help from advanced care providers or inform other incoming responders about the details of the situation found.

- Inside a hospital, a floor nurse may call a code to which a resuscitation team with appropriate equipment will respond. To be an effective BLS provider, you must understand your local protocols on how to call for additional help.

Knowledge Check

You are an EMS provider who has responded to a bystander report of a person who has collapsed. Your BLS assessment indicates cardiac arrest. Because you are the EMS response, to whom might you communicate about the arrest?

Chest Compressions

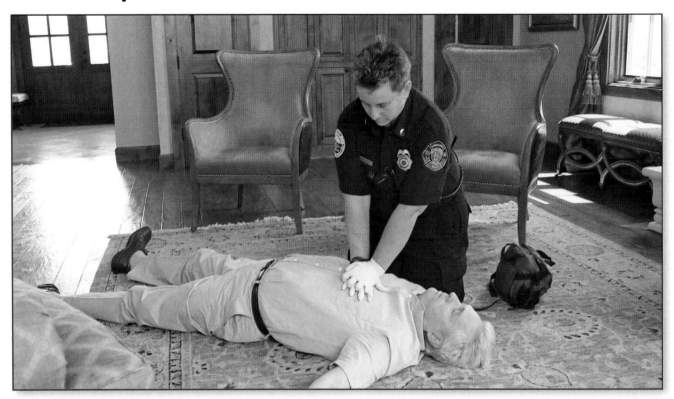

There are basic CPR skills used to provide the most effective approach to cardiac arrest.

These include the following:

- High-quality chest compressions
- High-quality rescue breaths using a CPR mask or bag-mask device
- Use of an automated external defibrillator
- Checking for life-threatening emergencies using a BLS assessment

External compression of the chest increases pressure inside the chest and directly compresses the heart, forcing blood to move from the chest to the lungs, heart, brain, and the rest of the body.

Focus on high-quality techniques:

- Compress deeply, more than 2 inches. It is likely you will not compress deep enough. While injury could occur from deeper compressions, do not let the fear of this affect compression depth.
- Compress fast, between 100 and 120 times per minute. Do not let a higher compression speed result in a shallower compression depth.
- Do not lean on the chest between compressions. Allow the chest wall to fully recoil, or rebound, at the top of each compression.
- Minimize interruptions when doing compressions. Blood pressure is created and maintained with ongoing compressions. When compressions stop, pressure is quickly lost and has to slowly be built up again.

CPR on a Firm Surface

Compression of the chest increases the internal pressure of the chest and heart, forcing blood out into other areas of the body. Placing a person on a firm surface is essential for compressions to be effective. If a person is on a soft surface, such as a mattress, compression of the chest is compromised.

Full Recoil of the Chest

Allowing the chest to fully return, or recoil, to its normal position at the top of each compression is a measure of high-quality compressions. Full recoil allows the heart to refill more completely between compressions and increases overall blood flow.

When compressing properly, you may hear and feel changes in the chest wall. This is normal. Forceful external chest compressions may cause chest injury but are critical if the person is to survive. Reassess your hand positioning and continue compressions.

As an alternative approach, you can grasp the wrist of one hand with the other when it is difficult to compress with the heels of both hands.

Compression Injury

Minor injury could result from deeper compressions. On an adult, this begins to occur at compression depths greater than 2.4 inches.

Children and Infants

The compression technique for a child is similar to that of adults, but less forceful. Push deep, straight down $1/3$ depth of the chest, or about 2 inches. For smaller children, the heel of one hand can be used to compress.

Compressions on a larger child can be tiring. If needed, use both hands to perform compressions.

When doing chest compressions on an infant with 2 or more providers, encircle the sides of the chest with your hands and use your thumb tips to compress the lower third of the breastbone. Push deep, at least $1/3$ depth of the chest or about $1^1/_2$ inches.

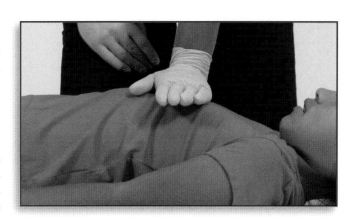

Knowledge Check

What are the 4 measures of high-quality chest compressions for an adult?

Chest Compressions

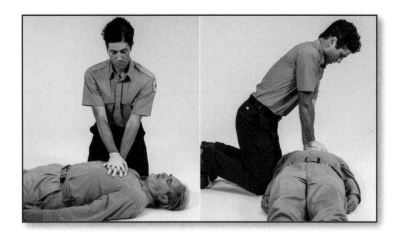

Adult

- Position person face up on a firm, flat surface. Kneel close to chest. Place heel of one hand on center of chest, on lower half of breastbone. Place heel of other hand on top of and parallel to first.
- Position your shoulders directly above your hands. Lock your elbows. Bending at waist, use upper body weight to push.
- Push deep, straight down at least 2 inches. Lift hands and allow chest to fully recoil. Move immediately into next compression. Compress fast, at a rate of 100–120 times per minute.

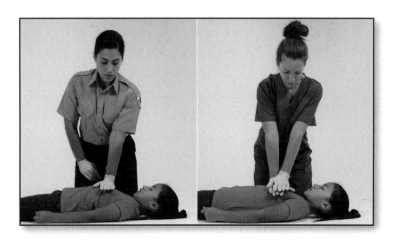

Child

- Position child face up on a firm, flat surface. Kneel close to chest. Place heel of one hand on lower half of breastbone, just above point where ribs meet.
- Position your shoulder directly above your hand. Lock your elbow. Bending at waist, use upper body weight to push.
- Push deep, straight down $1/3$ depth of chest, or about 2 inches. Lift hand and allow chest to fully recoil. Move immediately into next compression. Compress fast, at a rate of 100–120 times per minute.
- If needed, use 2 hands to compress.

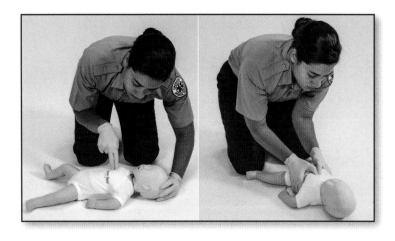

Infant

- Position infant face up on a firm, flat surface. Place 2 fingertips on breastbone just below nipple line.
- Push deep, at least $1/3$ depth of chest, or about $1\frac{1}{2}$ inches. Lift fingers and allow chest to fully recoil. Move immediately into next compression. Compress fast, at a rate of 100–120 times per minute.
- When doing chest compressions with 2 or more providers, encircle the sides of the chest with your hands and use your thumb tips to compress the lower third of the breastbone.

SKILL GUIDE 1

Rescue Breaths

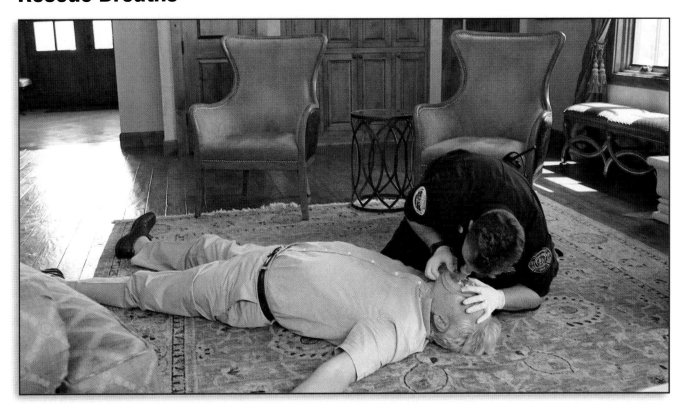

Rescue breaths are artificial breaths given to someone who is not breathing. They are given by blowing air into the mouth to inflate the lungs. The air you breathe contains about 21% oxygen. Your exhaled air still contains between 16% and 17% oxygen. This exhaled oxygen is enough to support someone's life.

Establishing an Airway

To give rescue breaths, you need to make sure there is an open airway. The airway is the only path for getting air into the lungs.

An unresponsive person can lose muscle tone. If flat on his or her back, the base of the tongue can relax and obstruct the airway. This is the most common cause of a blocked airway.

The tongue is attached to the lower jaw. Lifting the jaw forward pulls the tongue away from the back of the throat and opens the airway.

Head Tilt-Chin Lift

You can open a person's airway by using the head tilt-chin lift technique:

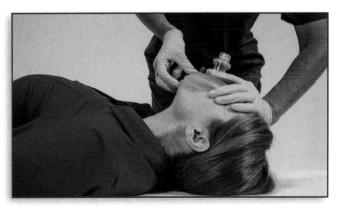

- Place one hand on the forehead.
- Place the fingertips of your other hand under the bony part of the chin.
- Apply firm, backward pressure on the forehead while lifting the chin upward. This will tilt the head back and move the jaw forward.
- Maintain the head tilt with your hand on the forehead. Leave the mouth slightly open.
- Avoid pressing into the soft tissue of the chin with your fingers, as this can also obstruct the airway.

Using a CPR Mask

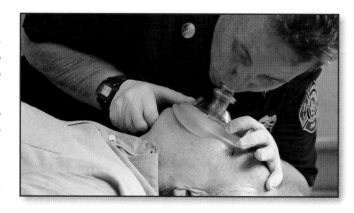

Although the risk is very low, as a BLS provider, use a protective barrier such as a CPR mask or bag-mask device when giving rescue breaths to minimize your exposure to infectious disease.

Each breath should be about 1 second in length and have only enough air to create a visible rise of the chest, but no more. Additional air is unnecessary.

Remove your mouth and let the person exhale between breaths. Take a regular breath before delivering the second rescue breath.

If you remove your hands from the head, the airway will close again. It is necessary to open the airway each time you give rescue breaths.

If you cannot get the chest to rise with a breath, reposition the head further back by using head tilt-chin lift again and try another breath.

Children and Infants

Rescue breaths for children and infants are performed in the same manner as for adults. It is recommended to use an appropriately sized pediatric CPR mask.

The airway of an infant may become blocked if the head is tilted too far. Position an infant's head in a neutral position, in which the ear openings are level with the infant's shoulders.

Special care should be taken not to give too much air in a single breath. Provide only enough air to make the chest visibly rise, but no more.

Giving Rescue Breaths without a Barrier Device

Depending on your relationship with someone or the availability of PPE, you may elect to perform rescue breaths without the use of a barrier device such as a CPR mask or bag mask. Mouth-to-mouth breaths can be given by pinching the nose, opening your mouth wide, and sealing your mouth around the person's mouth. Mouth-to-nose breaths can also be done by pressing the lips closed and sealing your mouth around the person's nose. With smaller children and infants, it may be necessary to seal your mouth around both the child's mouth and nose.

Laryngectomy

Some people breathe through a surgically created opening in the neck called a stoma. It is reasonable to use a round, pediatric CPR mask over the stoma to give rescue breaths. The stoma may still be connected to the normal airway. If air appears to be escaping through the mouth and nose, pinch the nose, close the mouth, and resume breaths through the stoma with the mask.

Gastric Inflation

Excessive air on rescue breaths can force air into the stomach. This can result in vomiting and complicate resuscitation efforts. Providing just enough air to create a visual rise of the chest, but no more, verifies a successful breath and minimizes the chance of forcing air into the stomach.

Cricoid Pressure

The use of cricoid pressure to prevent gastric inflation during rescue breaths is no longer recommended.

Jaw Thrust

The jaw thrust is a convenient airway technique, especially when working in a team or when using a bag-mask device. The provider is located above the person's head and uses 2 hands to tilt the head and thrust the jaw upward.

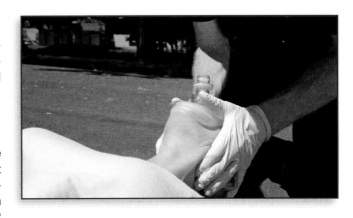

Using a Bag-Mask

A bag-mask device allows providers to provide rescue breaths without having to blow into a person's mouth. It can also deliver high concentrations of oxygen when connected to an oxygen delivery system. A bag-mask can be used by a single BLS provider but is best used by 2 providers.

Bag-mask rescue breaths for children or infants are done in the same manner as an adult. It is recommended that an appropriately sized pediatric bag-mask be used.

Oropharyngeal Airways (OPAs)

The use of an oropharyngeal airway (OPA) is recommended with the use of a bag-mask device to help maintain an open airway. Follow your local protocols on the use of OPAs.

Jaw Thrust without Head Tilt

When caring for someone who is seriously injured, establishing an open airway is a higher priority than protecting a possible injury to the spine. Without a patent airway a person will not survive, regardless of injury.

When the potential for a neck injury exists, a jaw thrust without head tilt can be used to open the airway.

If you find the jaw thrust without head tilt does not open the airway, use jaw thrust with head tilt, or the head tilt-chin lift technique, instead. You must establish an airway for a person to survive.

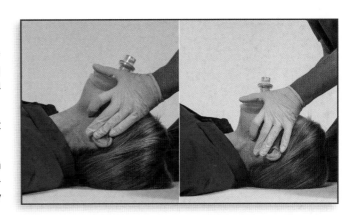

Knowledge Check

What is the recommended length and volume of a rescue breath?

Rescue Breaths Using a CPR Mask

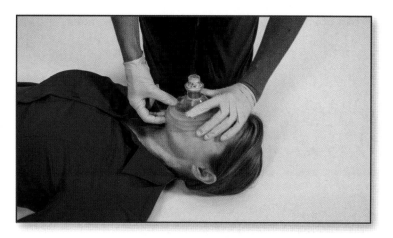

Position Mask

- Inspect mask to make sure one-way valve is in place.
- Place mask flat on person's face with top of mask over bridge of nose.
- Use thumb and forefinger to provide uniform pressure around top of mask.
- Use thumb of your hand lifting chin to control bottom.

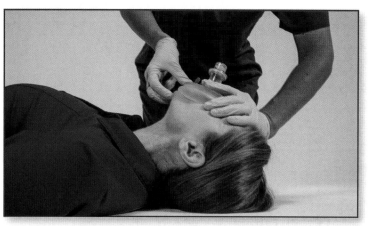

Establish Airway

- Hook fingertips of hand controlling bottom of mask under bony ridge of chin.
- Tilt head and lift chin to open airway. Lift face up into mask to create an airtight seal.

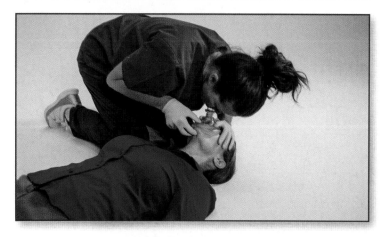

Deliver Breath

- Blow through valve opening to deliver breaths.
- Each breath is 1 second in length. Give only enough air to create a visible rise of chest, but no more.
- Remove mouth and let person exhale after each breath. Take a breath before delivering another rescue breath.

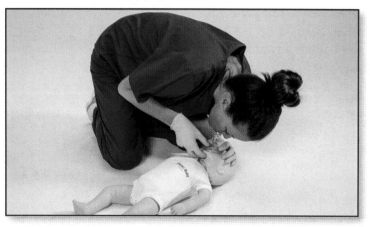

Children and Infants

- When possible, use appropriately sized mask.
- Be careful not to give too much air.

Jaw Thrust

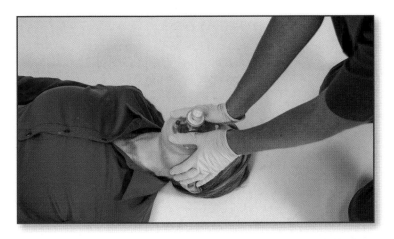

Place Mask

- Position yourself above person's head.
- Place mask flat on face with top over bridge of nose.
- Place thumbs and heels of hands along sides of mask to seal it to face.
- Hook index fingers under angles of jaw, just below ears.

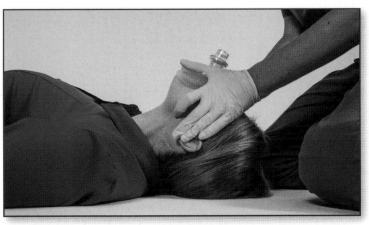

Establish Airway

- Lift and tilt head backwards.
- Lift jaw upward and into mask with index fingers using counter pressure against cheeks.

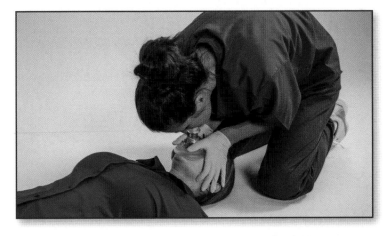

Deliver Breath

- Blow through valve opening to deliver breaths.
- Each breath is 1 second in length. Give only enough air to create a visible rise of chest, but no more.
- Remove mouth and let person exhale after each breath. Take a breath before delivering another rescue breath.

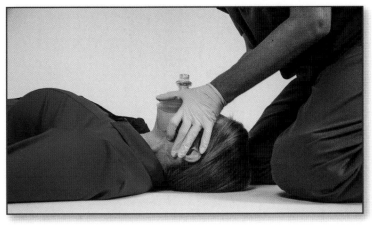

Jaw Thrust Without Head Tilt

- If you suspect a neck injury, use a jaw thrust without head tilt to open an airway.
- If you are unable to establish an airway this way, use jaw thrust with head tilt or head tilt–chin lift instead.

Rescue Breaths Using a Bag-Mask

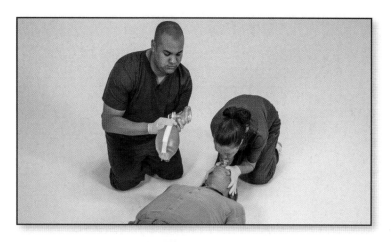

Prepare Bag-Mask

- If available, have another provider give rescue breaths with CPR mask until bag-mask is ready.
- Inspect bag-mask to make sure it is ready for use.

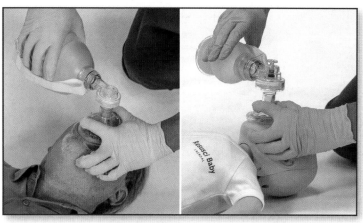

Place Mask/Establish Airway

- Positioning yourself above person's head, place mask flat on face with top over bridge of nose.
- Use thumb and index finger of hand in a C position to seal mask to face.
- Hook remaining fingers in an E position under bony ridge of chin.
- Tilt head and lift jaw up into mask to open airway.

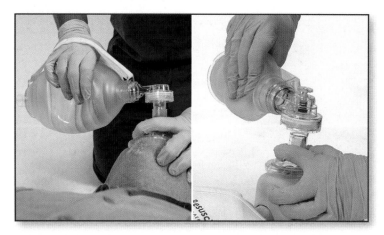

Deliver Rescue Breaths

- Squeeze bag with other hand to deliver breaths.
- Give each breath over 1 second; make chest visibly rise with each breath, but no more.

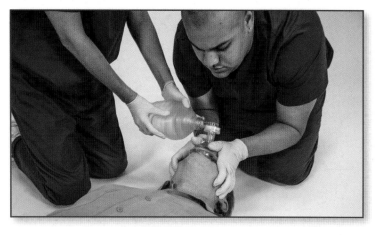

Using a Bag-Mask with 2 Providers

- Position yourself above the person's head.
- While a second provider holds bag, place mask on face and use jaw thrust to open airway.
- Have second provider squeeze bag with 2 hands to deliver breaths.
- Give each breath over 1 second; make chest visibly rise with each breath, but no more.

SKILL GUIDE 4

Automated External Defibrillation

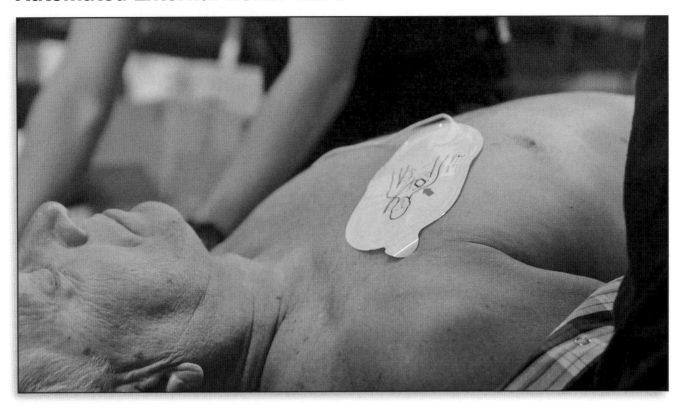

AEDs are designed to be simple to operate. Voice instructions, lights, and screen prompts guide an operator through use.

Public Access Defibrillation

Public access defibrillation (PAD) programs promote bystander training, access, and use of AEDs, especially in locations where large numbers of people may gather such as airports, stores, hotels, gyms, and convention centers.

There are many different brands of AEDs, but the same basic steps for operation apply to all.

Turn on the AED. Opening the lid will turn on the power for some AEDs. With others, simply press the power button. This starts voice instructions and readies the device for use.

Adhere defibrillation pads to chest. Pads must be applied to a bare chest. If needed, quickly tear away or use scissors to remove all clothing from the torso. Dry the chest quickly if wet. For a woman, remove the bra to provide better access for pad placement.

Locate and pull out the defibrillation pads. The pads have pictures on them to show proper placement. Proper placement will assure that the pads are able to direct the electrical shock through the heart. Peel the pads from the backing sheet one at a time and place each as shown in the pictures. Place one pad below the right collarbone, above the nipple, and beside the breastbone. Make sure it adheres well by pressing it flat. Place the other pad lower on the left side, over the ribs, and a few inches below the armpit. Again, press firmly.

Allow the AED to analyze the heart rhythm. Most AEDs automatically start analyzing once the pads are in place. Stop CPR. Movement can interrupt the analysis. Be certain that no one is touching the person. If defibrillation is advised, the AED will begin to charge for shock delivery.

Deliver a shock if directed by the AED. To prevent the accidental shock of a provider, quickly look to make sure no one, including you, is in contact with the person before delivering the shock. For most AEDs, a button is pressed to deliver the shock. Once a shock has been delivered, immediately resume CPR starting with chest compressions.

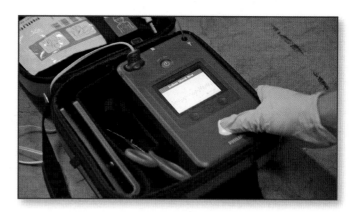

In cases when a shock is not indicated by the AED, immediately resume CPR. Voice instructions and additional analysis by the AED guides you through further care.

If a person responds, stop CPR and place him or her in a recovery position. Leave the AED turned on and pads attached in case cardiac arrest occurs again.

Automatic Shock Delivery

Some AEDs deliver a shock automatically after charging. An accidental shock can be prevented by making sure no one is in contact with the person being defibrillated.

AED Maintenance

An AED needs to be maintained in order to be ready any time a cardiac arrest could occur. AEDs have built-in self-testing functions and indicators to verify readiness. Batteries and pads have expiration dates for use. Additional supplies such as scissors, razors, towels, and gloves may need to be accounted for. Always follow the manufacturer's instructions for maintenance.

Children and Infants

Cardiac arrests involving children are likely caused by the initial loss of the airway or breathing. High-quality CPR with effective rescue breaths may be the only treatment required for successful resuscitation.

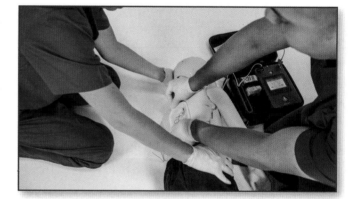

However, conditions can occur for which defibrillation of a child or infant is warranted. Most AEDs have specially designed pads or mechanisms available that reduce the defibrillation energy to a level more appropriate for a smaller body size.

The steps for using an AED on a child or infant are similar to an adult. For smaller children and infants, place one pad on the center of the chest just below the collarbones. Attach the second pad on the center of the back between the shoulder blades.

If an AED specifically equipped for use on a child or infant is not available, an AED configured for an adult can be used instead.

Manual Defibrillator Preferred for Infants

If available, and you are trained in its use, a manual defibrillator, in which the energy dose is adjustable, is preferred for defibrillation of an infant.

AED Troubleshooting

AEDs are also designed to detect problems during use and guide you through corrective actions. If a troubleshooting message occurs at any time, stay calm and follow the AED voice instructions.

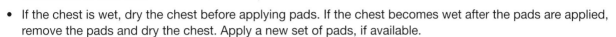

When it becomes necessary to troubleshoot an AED, CPR should be provided, without interruption, until the problem is corrected or another AED becomes available. Pauses of CPR lasting longer than 10 seconds should be avoided.

- If the AED indicates a problem with the pads, the pads are not completely adhered to the skin or there is a poor connection to the AED. Press pads firmly, especially in the center, to make sure they are adhering well. Make sure the pads' cable connector is firmly connected to the AED.

- If the chest is wet, dry the chest before applying pads. If the chest becomes wet after the pads are applied, remove the pads and dry the chest. Apply a new set of pads, if available.

- Thick chest hair may prevent the AED pads from adhering to the skin. If chest hair is excessive, quickly shave the hair in the areas where the pads will be placed. If pads were placed over chest hair and do not adhere, pull the pads off quickly and shave the hair. Attach another set of pads, if available. Otherwise, reapply the original pads.

- Another troubleshooting message may indicate that analysis has been interrupted due to movement. Stop all sources of movement, such as chest compressions or rescue breaths.

- If a message indicates the need to replace a battery, there may be only enough energy for a limited number of shocks and only a few more minutes of operation. If the AED fails to operate, the depleted battery should be removed and replaced with a new one. If a battery needs replacement during resuscitation, it should be replaced during a CPR interval.

- A person should be removed from standing water before using an AED. It is okay to use an AED when a person is lying on a wet surface, such as in the rain or near a swimming pool. An AED should never be immersed in water or have fluids spilled on it.

- AEDs can also be used safely on metal surfaces, such as gratings or stairwells. Make sure pads do not directly touch any metal surface.

- Someone may have a surgically implanted device in the chest, such as a pacemaker or an automated internal defibrillator. A noticeable lump and surgical scar will be visible. If the implanted device is in the way of correct pad placement, place the pads so the edges are at least 1 inch away from the device.

- Defibrillating over medication patches could reduce the effectiveness of the shock. If a medication patch is interfering with placement, use a gloved hand to peel off the patch and wipe away any remaining residue before placing pads.

Knowledge Check

You have responded to a person in cardiac arrest. CPR is already in progress. You kneel next to the man and lay the AED next to his head. What are the 4 basic steps you will take to use the AED on him?

Using an AED — Adult

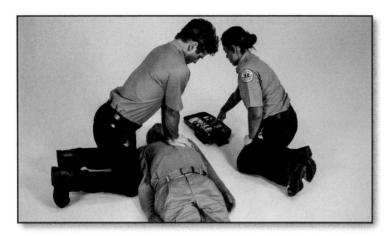

Perform CPR

- If your BLS assessment indicates cardiac arrest, perform CPR.

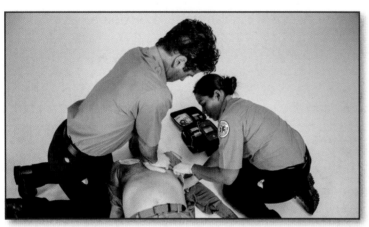

When Available, Attach AED Immediately

- Turn on AED and bare person's chest.
- Peel first pad from backing and place below right collarbone, above nipple, and beside breastbone.
- Remove second pad from backing and place on left side, over ribs, and a few inches below armpit.

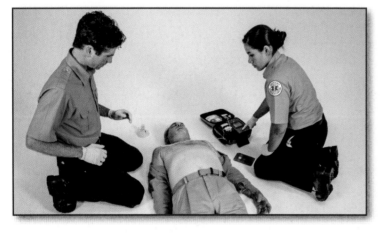

If Indicated, Deliver Shock

- Allow AED to analyze heart. Stop CPR. Do not touch the person.
- If shock is advised, clear everyone and press button to deliver shock.

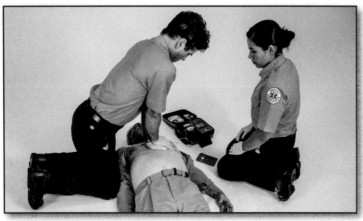

Resume CPR

- Quickly resume CPR starting with chest compressions. Follow any additional voice instructions from AED.
- Continue until another BLS provider takes over, the person shows signs of life, or you are too exhausted to continue.
- If person responds, stop CPR and place in recovery position. Leave AED on and attached.

Using an AED — Children and Infants

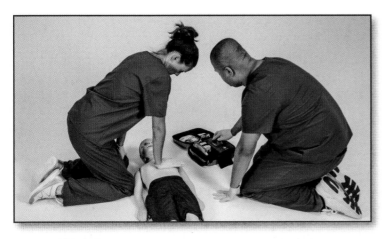

Perform CPR

- If your BLS assessment indicates cardiac arrest, perform CPR.

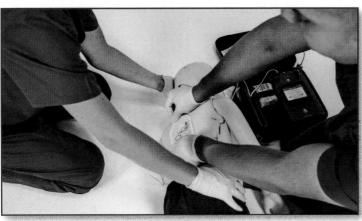

When Available, Attach AED Immediately

- Turn on AED and bare child's chest.
- Peel first pad from backing and place in center of chest just below collarbones.
- Roll child and place second pad on center of back between shoulder blades.

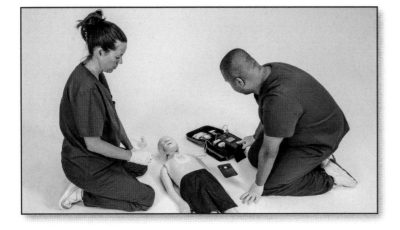

If Indicated, Deliver Shock

- Allow AED to analyze heart. Stop CPR. Do not touch the child.
- If shock is advised, clear everyone and press button to deliver shock.

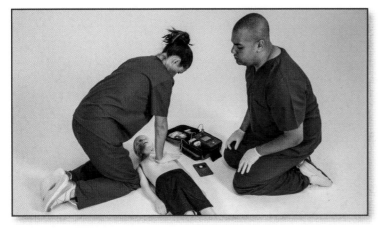

Resume CPR

- Quickly resume CPR starting with chest compressions. Follow any additional voice instructions from AED.
- Continue until another BLS provider takes over, the child shows signs of life, or you are too exhausted to continue.
- If child responds, stop CPR and place in recovery position. Leave AED on and attached.

BLS Assessment

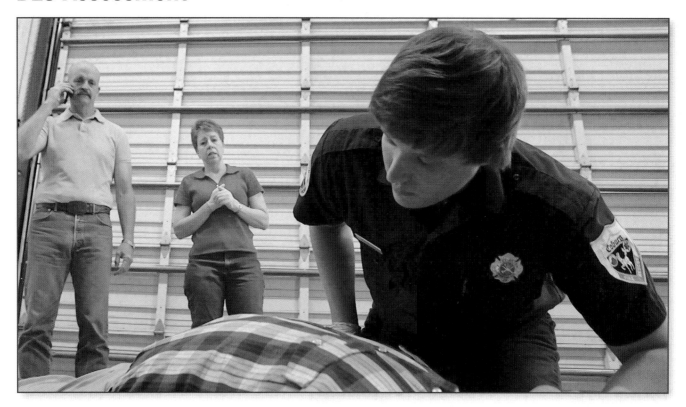

The BLS assessment is a simple way to quickly identify if resuscitation is required. It is the same for all ages and is performed quickly.

Ensure the scene is safe. Before anything else, pause and assess the scene for hazards. If the scene is not safe, do not enter until hazards have been minimized or eliminated. Take standard precautions to prevent contact with blood or other potentially infectious materials.

Assess responsiveness. If it is safe, check for responsiveness. Tap or squeeze the person's shoulder and ask loudly, "Are you all right?" For an infant, tap the foot.

Assess for breathing and pulse. If unresponsive, quickly look at the person's chest and face for signs of normal breathing. At the same time check for a pulse.

Normal breathing is effortless, quiet, and regular. Weak, irregular gasping, snorting, or gurgling sounds, known as agonal breaths, can occur early in cardiac arrest. These actions provide no usable oxygen. This is not normal breathing.

Check the carotid pulse in the neck. Take at least 5 but no longer than 10 seconds to assess breathing and pulse. If you are unsure, assume they are absent.

Activate the emergency response protocol for your setting and get an AED. If not already being done, tell another person to activate the protocol and get an AED. Relay what you have found so it can be passed on.

Checking Pulses

Locate the bony Adam's apple with your fingers. Slide them into the groove between the windpipe and the muscle on the side of the neck closest to you. For a child, check the carotid pulse or femoral pulse in the leg. Place your fingers just below the middle of the crease where the leg and torso meet. For infants, feel for the brachial pulse on the inside of the upper arm. Lay your fingers across the arm and compress inward.

Activating Additional Resources

The need to activate additional resources is an important part of the BLS assessment. Unlike lay providers, who simply need to activate emergency medical services (EMS), the additional resources needed by BLS providers can vary, depending on the circumstance. In most cases, the actions to take are already established through emergency response protocols. Because of this, the point at which you activate additional resources in a BLS assessment is highly dependent on the situation and your local protocols.

When Alone

If you are alone and have witnessed a sudden collapse, activate your emergency response protocol and get an AED yourself. Quickly return to the person. This action is the same regardless of the age of the person.

If you are alone and did not witness the collapse, or you highly suspect a secondary cause such as drowning, suffocation, or opioid overdose, provide about 2 minutes of CPR before leaving to activate your protocol and get an AED yourself. This is the most likely situation encountered with children.

Modification for Drowning

Due to the hypoxic nature of drowning, the BLS assessment is modified slightly. Once a person is removed from the water, immediately assess for normal breathing and pulse. If breathing is absent or only gasping, provide 2 initial rescue breaths that make the chest visibly rise. If the pulse is clearly felt continue with rescue breathing. If a pulse is absent, or if you are not certain, begin CPR. Attach an AED as soon as one is available.

Your assessment of the person and situation will determine the care you provide. If the person is breathing normally, and uninjured, place him or her in a side-lying recovery position.

If the person is not breathing or only gasping, but definitely has a pulse, he or she is in respiratory arrest. The indicated care is rescue breathing, which is ongoing rescue breaths provided without chest compressions.

If the person is not breathing, or only gasping, and does not have a pulse, he or she is in cardiac arrest. The indicated care is CPR, a repeating combination of chest compressions and rescue breaths.

Recovery Position

The recovery position helps protect the airway by using gravity to drain fluids from the mouth and keep the tongue from blocking the airway.

Frequently assess and monitor the person's breathing. The condition can quickly become worse and require additional care.

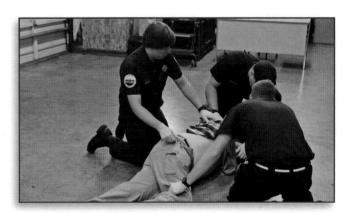

Knowledge Check

You have responded to someone complaining of severe pressure in the chest. As you are talking to the person, he suddenly slumps onto the floor. You kneel next to him, squeeze his shoulder, and loudly ask, "Are you all right?" He is unresponsive, so you look closely at the face and chest for breathing and feel for a carotid pulse; he makes a brief gasping snort, but then remains still. You cannot feel a pulse within 10 seconds. What do you do next?

BLS Assessment

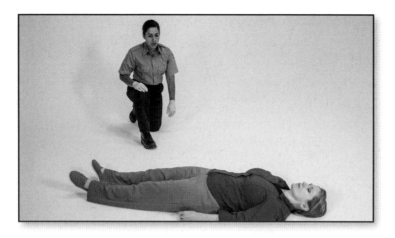

Assess Scene

- Pause and assess scene for safety.
- If unsafe, or if it becomes unsafe at any time, GET OUT!

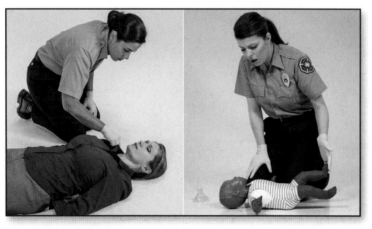

Check for Response

- Tap or squeeze shoulder and ask loudly, "Are you all right?"
- For an infant, tap the foot.
- If alone, shout out for help.
- Position person face-up on a firm, flat surface.

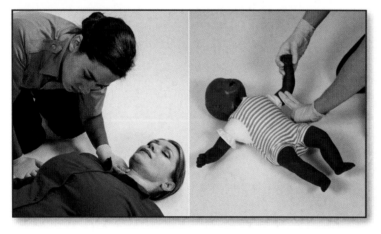

Check Breathing and Pulse

- Look at face and chest for normal breathing. If unsure, assume breathing is not normal.
- Weak, irregular gasping, snorting, or gurgling is not normal breathing.
- At same time check for a carotid pulse. For infant, check brachial pulse.
- Take at least 5 seconds and no longer than 10 to check breathing and pulse.

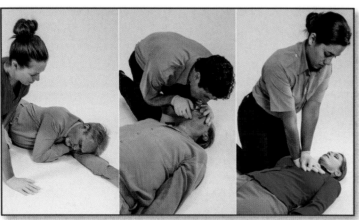

Provide Indicated Care

- If not already done, activate emergency response protocol and get an AED.
- No response, with normal breathing and pulse? Place in recovery position.
- No response with breathing absent and pulse present? Begin rescue breathing.
- No response with normal breathing and pulse absent? Begin CPR.

Recovery Position

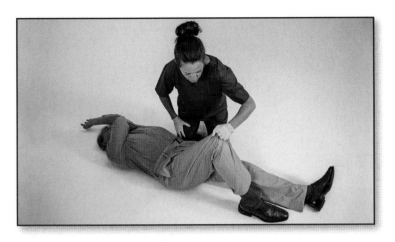

Prepare

- Place arm nearest you up alongside head.
- Bring far arm across chest and place back of hand against cheek.
- Grasp far leg just above knee and pull it up so the foot is flat on ground.

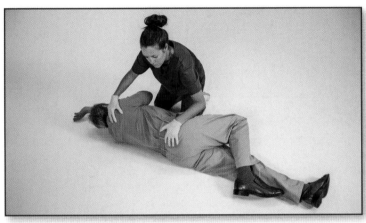

Roll

- Grasping shoulder and hip, roll person toward you in a single motion, keeping head, shoulders, and body from twisting.
- Roll far enough for face to be angled toward ground.

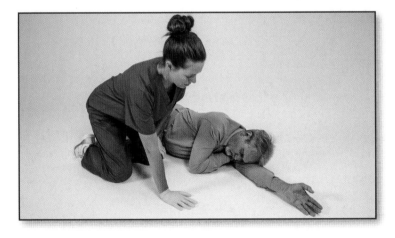

Stabilize

- Position elbow and legs to stabilize head and body. Ensure there is no pressure on chest that restricts breathing.
- Make sure head ends up resting on extended arm and head, neck, and body are aligned.
- If person has been seriously injured, do not place in a recovery position unless fluids are in airway, or you need to leave to get help.

Caring for Respiratory Arrest

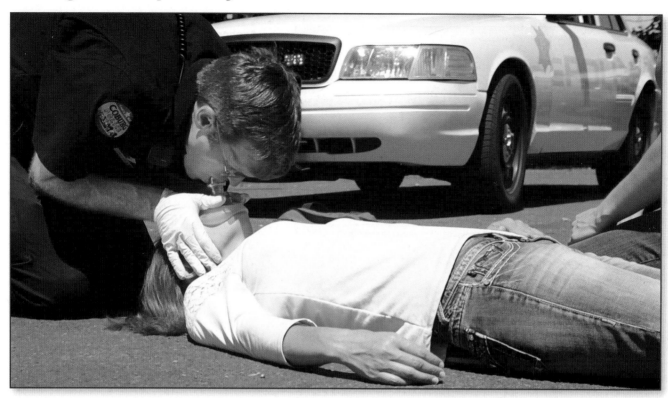

A person in respiratory arrest has stopped breathing but still has a beating heart. Without immediate intervention, respiratory arrest can quickly progress to cardiac arrest. Rescue breathing is the treatment for respiratory arrest. For an adult, provide 1 high-quality rescue breath every 5 to 6 seconds or about 10 to 12 breaths per minute.

Reassess the pulse about every 2 minutes. Take no longer than 10 seconds to do so. If the pulse is absent and tissue signs indicate poor perfusion, or you are unsure, perform CPR, starting with compressions.

If an opioid overdose is suspected, consider the use of naloxone as indicated by your local protocols.

Children and Infants

The rate of rescue breaths when performing rescue breathing for children and infants is 1 breath every 3 to 5 seconds, or about 12 to 20 breaths per minute. When monitoring the pulse of an infant, check for the brachial pulse.

Add compressions and perform CPR on a child or infant if the pulse rate is 60 beats per minute or fewer and it appears the heart is too weak to adequately move blood forward.

Signs of poor blood perfusion include the following:

- Pale, mottled, or bluish skin
- Weak pulse
- Cool extremity temperature

Knowledge Check

You respond to a teenager who was found unresponsive. Your BLS assessment indicates she is not breathing, but you can clearly feel her carotid pulse. Describe the care you will provide for her.

Caring for Respiratory Arrest — Adult

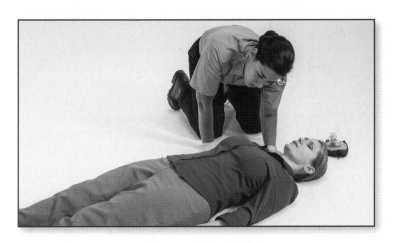

Assess

- If safe, tap or squeeze shoulder. Ask loudly, "Are you all right?" **No response!**
- Check face and chest for normal breathing. Check pulse at same time. **Normal breathing absent! Pulse present!**
- Activate emergency response protocol to get additional help and an AED.

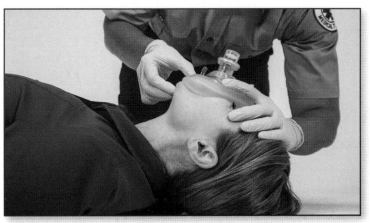

Establish an Airway

- Use head tilt-chin lift or jaw thrust to open airway.
- If you suspect neck injury, use jaw thrust without head tilt.

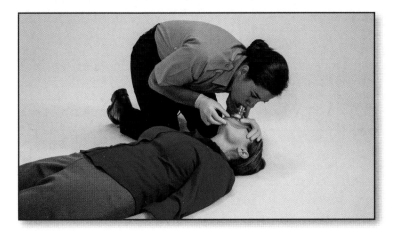

Give Rescue Breaths

- Provide 1 rescue breath every 5-6 seconds, or 10-12 times per minute.
- Give each breath over 1 second; make chest visibly rise with each breath, but no more.
- Reassess pulse every 2 minutes, taking no longer than 10 seconds to do so.
- Continue until another BLS provider takes over, the person shows signs of life, or you are too exhausted to continue.

Caring for Respiratory Arrest — Children and Infants

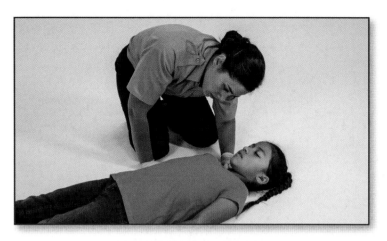

Assess Child or Infant

- If safe, tap or squeeze shoulder. Ask loudly, "Are you all right?" For an infant, tap the foot and shout loudly. *No response!*
- Check face and chest for normal breathing. Check pulse at same time. For an infant, check the brachial pulse. *Normal breathing absent! Pulse present!*
- Activate emergency response protocol to get additional help and an AED.

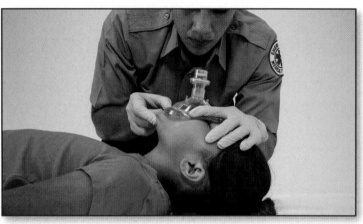

Establish an Airway

- Use head tilt-chin lift or jaw thrust to open airway.
- If you suspect neck injury, use jaw thrust without head tilt.

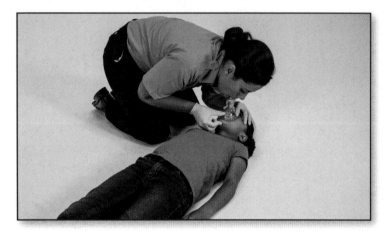

Give Rescue Breaths

- Provide 1 rescue breath every 3-5 seconds, or 12-20 times per minute.
- Give each breath over 1 second; make chest visibly rise with each breath, but no more.
- Reassess pulse every 2 minutes, taking no longer than 10 seconds to do so.
- Continue until another BLS provider takes over, the person shows signs of life, or you are too exhausted to continue

Caring for Cardiac Arrest

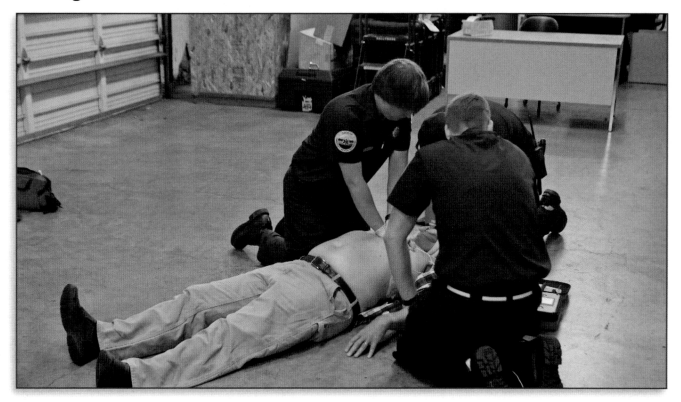

Immediate, high-quality CPR and defibrillation with an AED can double or even triple the chance for survival from sudden cardiac arrest.

CPR combines both chest compressions and rescue breaths to provide a limited amount of oxygen to the brain and vital organs of someone in cardiac arrest.

CPR buys more time in which defibrillation can work and helps make the heart more receptive to defibrillation.

The ratio of chest compressions to rescue breaths used in an adult CPR cycle is 30:2. Cycles of compressions and breaths are repeated without stopping.

Keep interruptions to compressions as short as possible. Take less than 10 seconds to give rescue breaths.

Use the AED immediately when it arrives. Turn on the AED and adhere the defibrillation pads to the bare chest. Allow the AED to analyze the heart. If a shock is advised, make sure you are not touching the person before delivering the shock.

Immediately after a shock is delivered, resume CPR starting with compressions. Voice instructions and additional analysis by the AED will guide you through further care. Don't stop until the person shows signs of life, another BLS provider takes over, or you are too exhausted to continue.

If the person begins to breathe, move, or respond, stop CPR and place the person in the recovery position. Leave the AED turned on and pads attached in case cardiac arrest reoccurs. In cases where a shock is not indicated by the AED, immediately resume CPR. Continue to follow the AED's instructions.

When performing CPR, do the best you can. A person without breathing or circulation will not survive without help. Nothing you do can make the outcome worse.

Baring the Chest

When initiating CPR, it can be helpful to bare the chest in order to help with proper hand placement for compressions. When using an AED, it is necessary to bare the chest to place defibrillation pads.

Minimizing Pre-Shock and Post-Shock Interruptions

Minimizing any interruption to chest compressions is a defined goal for high-quality CPR. When 2 or more providers are available, shorten the pause immediately before a defibrillation shock by continuing chest compressions while pads are being placed. After a shock is delivered, immediately resume compressions, even before the AED voice prompt instructs you to.

Compression-Only CPR

Compression-only CPR is being widely promoted to people who are not trained in CPR in order to encourage and increase the chance for bystander care. Simple instructions in compression-only CPR are being shared through things such as social media and public service announcements. EMS dispatchers are also providing compression-only instructions during emergency calls.

Compression-only CPR is a limited approach to treating cardiac arrest. At some point, rescue breaths are essential for all cardiac arrests, especially for secondary cardiac arrest.

As a trained BLS provider, perform both compressions and breaths during CPR.

Children and Infants

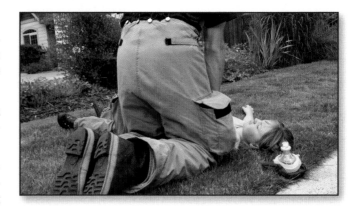

Most arrests involving children are secondary to the initial loss of an airway or breathing. Immediate CPR with an emphasis on effective rescue breaths may provide the only chance for survival.

The ratio of chest compressions to rescue breaths for a child or infant is 30:2. When there are more than 2 providers, the ratio is 15:2.

If an AED becomes available, use it immediately. It is unlikely that a child or infant will require defibrillation. Be prepared to immediately resume CPR if the AED does not advise a shock.

Knowledge Check

You responded to a man who collapsed. Your BLS assessment indicates cardiac arrest. You are with another BLS provider and have an AED with you. Describe the care you will provide for him.

BLS CARE

Caring for Cardiac Arrest — Adults

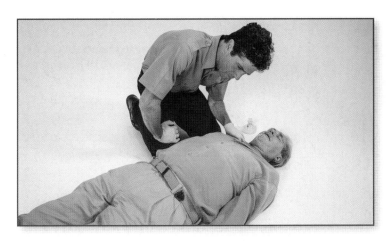

Assess Person

- If safe, tap or squeeze shoulder. Ask loudly, "Are you all right?" **No response!**
- Check face and chest for normal breathing. Check pulse at same time. **Normal breathing absent! Pulse absent!**
- Activate emergency response protocol to get additional help and an AED.

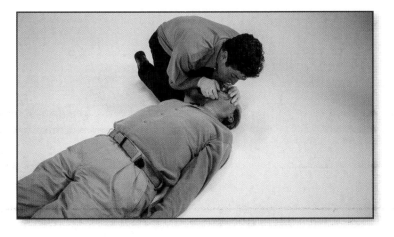

Give 30 Compressions

- Place heel of one hand on center of chest on the lower half of the breastbone. Place heel of other hand on top of first.
- Bring body up and over chest. Use upper body weight to push down deep, at least 2 inches.
- Push fast, at a rate of 100-120 times per minute. Allow chest to fully recoil.

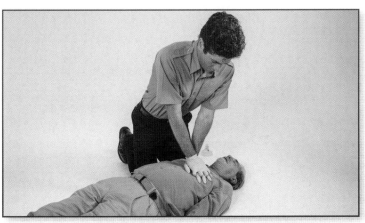

Give 2 Rescue Breaths

- Using a barrier device, establish an airway.
- Make chest visibly rise with each breath, but no more.
- Take a breath between rescue breaths. Give breaths in less than 10 seconds.
- Provide continuous cycles of 30 compressions and 2 rescue breaths.

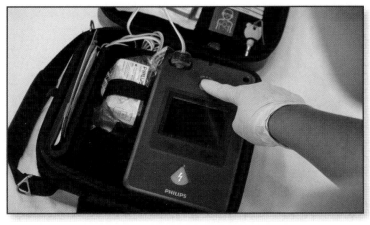

Use an AED

- If AED becomes available, stop CPR and use it immediately. Turn AED on and follow its voice instructions.
- Deliver a shock if indicated by AED. Immediately resume CPR after a shock is delivered or no shock is advised.
- Continue until another BLS provider takes over, the person shows signs of life, or you are too exhausted to continue.

Caring for Cardiac Arrest — Children

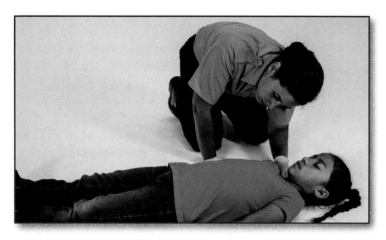

Assess Child

- If safe, tap or squeeze shoulder. Ask loudly, "Are you all right?" *No response!*
- Check face and chest for normal breathing. Check pulse at same time. *Normal breathing absent! Pulse absent!*
- Activate emergency response protocol to get additional help and an AED.

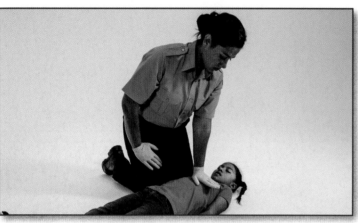

Give 30 Compressions

- Place heel of one hand on lower half of breastbone, just above point where ribs meet. Use both hands if needed.
- Bring body up and over chest. Use upper body weight to push down at least $1/3$ depth of the chest or about 2 inches.
- Push fast, at a rate of 100-120 times per minute. Allow chest to fully recoil.

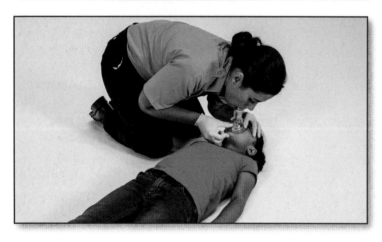

Give 2 Rescue Breaths

- Using a barrier device, establish an airway.
- Make chest visibly rise with each breath, but no more.
- Take a breath between rescue breaths. Give breaths in less than 10 seconds.
- Provide continuous cycles of 30 compressions and 2 rescue breaths.
- Continue until another BLS provider takes over, the person shows signs of life, or you are too exhausted to continue.

Caring for Cardiac Arrest — Infants

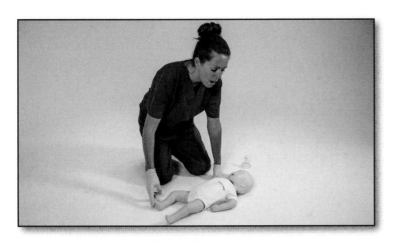

Assess Infant

- If safe, tap foot. Ask loudly, "Are you all right?" **No response!**
- Check face and chest for normal breathing. Check pulse at same time. **Normal breathing absent! Pulse absent!**
- Activate emergency response protocol to get additional help and an AED.

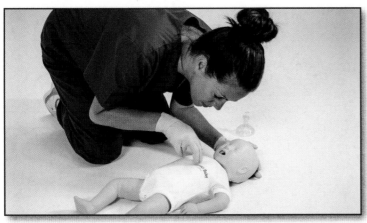

Give 30 Compressions

- Place 2 fingertips on breastbone just below nipple line.
- Compress at least $1/3$ depth of chest, or about $1\frac{1}{2}$ inches.
- Push fast, at a rate of 100–120 times per minute. Allow chest to fully recoil.

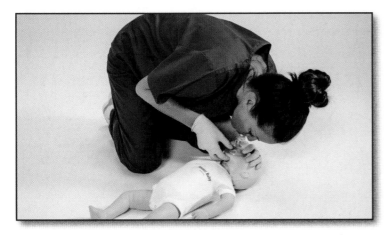

Give 2 Rescue Breaths

- Using a barrier device, establish an airway.
- Make chest visibly rise with each breath, but no more.
- Take a breath between rescue breaths. Give breaths in less than 10 seconds.
- Provide continuous cycles of 30 compressions and 2 rescue breaths.
- Continue until another BLS provider takes over, the person shows signs of life, or you are too exhausted to continue.

Multiple Provider Approach to CPR

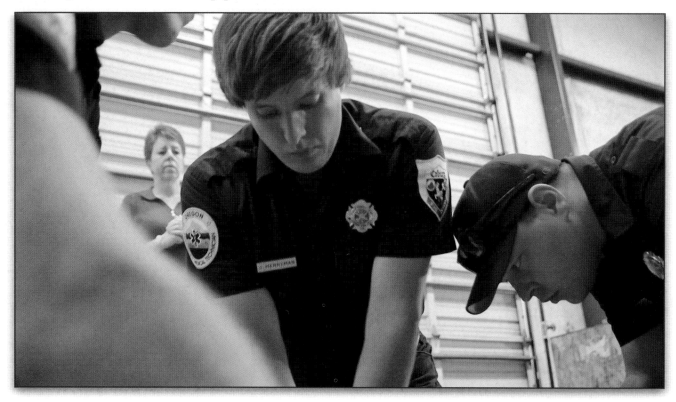

High-performance CPR not only requires high-quality CPR skills, but it also relies on the efficiency of multiple providers working as a team.

It is common for multiple providers to respond to a cardiac arrest but a resuscitation may start with a single provider. Other providers can be integrated as they arrive.

Counting Compressions

Counting compressions out loud is helpful to communicate and coordinate with others as a part of high-performance CPR.

Splitting Compressions and Breaths

When 2 providers are available to perform CPR, one performs chest compressions while the other gives rescue breaths. For adults, the ratio remains at 30 compressions and 2 rescue breaths.

The compressor pauses to allow rescue breaths to be given. Give breaths as quickly as possible to minimize the interruption.

Switching

High-quality compressions are tiring. Before an AED is attached, switch compressors every 2 minutes after rescue breaths at the end of a CPR cycle. Clearly communicate the details of a switch ahead of time to prevent confusion.

If a third provider is available, have him or her relieve the compressor while rescue breaths are being given to shorten the interruption.

Once an AED is attached, switch compressors during the pause in CPR when the AED reanalyzes the heart. This typically occurs every 2 minutes.

Children and Infants

With 2 CPR providers, use a 15-to-2 ratio of compressions and breaths for a child or infant. To accommodate the small size of an infant, encircle the sides of the chest with your hands and use your thumb tips to compress the lower third of the breastbone. Use a jaw thrust with either a CPR mask or bag mask to give rescue breaths.

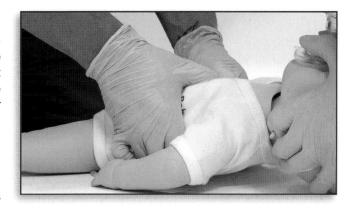

Team Approach

When 2 or more BLS providers respond in an emergency, orchestrating actions, much like a pit crew in a car race, is necessary for high-performance resuscitation.

Effective team communication is essential. Speak calmly and in simple terms. Ensure the person you are talking to understands. If you are asked to do something, repeat it back to confirm and reinforce the instructions.

It is important to recognize the common roles identified for a team resuscitation and be ready to assume any one of them.

- The compressor is typically the initial responding provider. A BLS assessment is done and CPR is started, beginning with compressions.
- When a second person is available, he or she becomes the ventilator and takes responsibility for maintaining an airway and giving rescue breaths.
- The team leader takes charge and maintains a general perspective to supervise and improve overall team performance. This person is also the main point of internal and external communication.
- An AED operator brings and quickly attaches defibrillation pads without interrupting CPR. He or she is also responsible for the efficient and safe delivery of defibrillation shocks.

Other roles may be filled as necessary—a second ventilator to help with the use of bag-mask, or a scribe or reporter to document patient information, treatments, and intervention times. In the transition to more advanced care, additional roles for actions such as administering medications may be added.

When an AED is attached, plan to relieve the compressor during the time an AED analyzes the heart. This typically occurs every 2 minutes. After a shock is delivered, or no shock is indicated, the new compressor immediately resumes CPR starting with compressions.

Communication within a Team

Closed loop communication is recommended when working in teams. Ensure you have the attention of the person to whom you are giving an instruction. Make sure the person understands the instruction. When you are instructed to do something, repeat the instruction back to the person to confirm your understanding. When you have finished doing what you have been asked, inform the person who asked you to do it.

Chest Compression Fraction (CCF)

Chest compression fraction is the percentage of overall CPR time that compressions are being performed. Higher percentages are associated with high-quality CPR and greater rates of survival for cardiac arrest. A fraction percentage of at least 60% is recommended, but much higher percentages are achievable.

Debriefing

After a resuscitation, a facilitated group discussion, or debriefing, lets team members reflect on the care provided. Debriefing identifies issues with skills, equipment, or established procedures. It also emphasizes and reinforces what was done well. Changes based on debriefing can improve the overall standard of care for future resuscitations. Using realistic, scenario-based practices is an excellent way to prepare for team-based resuscitations. Practice using a team approach.

Advanced Airways

An advanced airway device may be inserted into the throat during a resuscitation to protect and maintain an open airway. When an advanced airway device is in place, the mask from the bag-mask is removed and the bag is attached directly to the device to ventilate. As with other approaches to rescue breaths, provide only enough air to make the chest visibly rise.

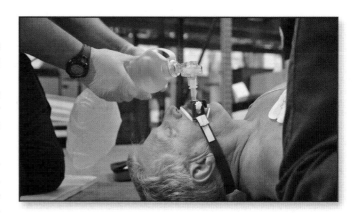

Once an advanced airway device is in place, it is no longer necessary to pause compressions to give breaths. Provide continuous compressions at a rate of 100 to 120 per minute. Regardless of age, provide a single breath every 6 seconds, or 10 times per minute.

Advanced Airways

An advanced airway is a device placed into the trachea or esophagus to allow direct ventilation into the lungs while helping to prevent aspiration of fluids or foreign material. Common airways include the laryngeal mask airway, supraglottic airway device, and endotracheal tube.

Knowledge Check

True or false? When 2 or more providers are available to perform CPR (assuming others are available to handle priority things such as getting an AED), split the compressions and breaths between providers.

Two-Provider CPR

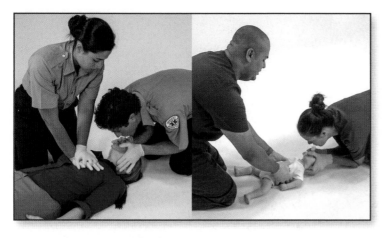

Coordination

- One provider delivers compressions while a second provider delivers rescue breaths.
- Avoid positioning both providers on the same side.
- Compressor pauses to allow for rescue breaths. Minimize pause as much as possible.

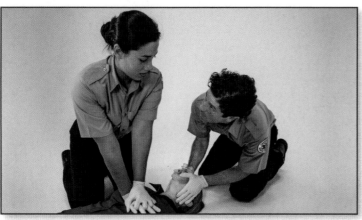

Preparing to Switch Compressors

- Compressions are tiring. Switch out compressor every 2 minutes.
- Clearly communicate ahead of time so everyone understands when the switch will occur.

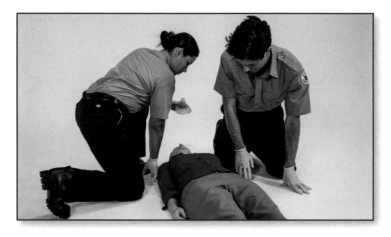

Switching

- Compressor moves towards the person's head during rescue breaths and prepares to become the new ventilator.
- Ventilator quickly moves to side of person's chest and begins compressions within 5 seconds.
- New ventilator gives rescue breaths at end of CPR cycle.

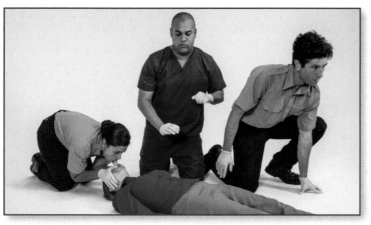

More Than 2 Providers

- If available, rotate extra providers into compressor role instead of ventilator.

High-Performance CPR Practice

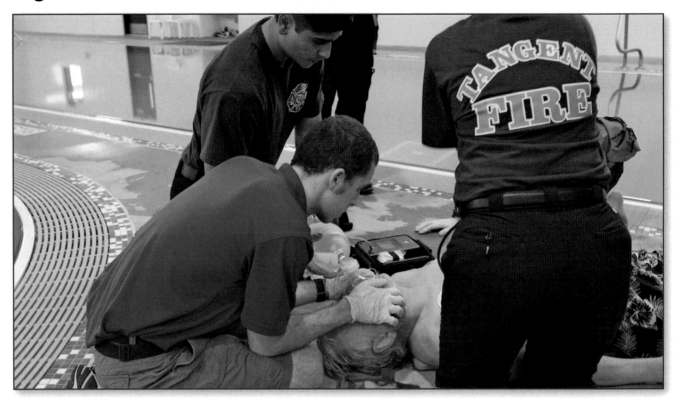

Now that you have learned and practiced all of your individual skills and treatments, you will act as a member of a BLS team in a mock resuscitation. This practice is intended to simulate, as much as possible, a real medical emergency.

There will be no guidance from your instructor. Simply apply your skills as best you can, given the circumstances. It is likely errors will occur, but you will have a chance to see how debriefing allows you to acknowledge them and make corrections for future resuscitations.

This practice will begin with the arrival of an AED and two-provider CPR already in progress. Your team will have at least 3 providers and the practice will continue until each team member has performed compressions for at least 2 minutes.

Your instructor will fill you in on any additional instructions and equipment you will be using.

Here are some things to keep in mind:

- Communicate! Talk about changes up front, before they occur.
- Have a single person in charge.
- Stay calm and help each other. Do not stop!
- Keep interruptions to compressions as short as possible.
- Once an AED is attached, switch compressors each time the AED analyzes, which typically occurs every 2 minutes.

High-Performance CPR Scenarios

Below are the situations that have occurred:

Adult Scenario: You arrive at a retirement center as part of an EMS response to a reported cardiac arrest of a 64-year-old man in the lobby. A BLS engine crew is already performing two-provider CPR. You and your crew are bringing in an AED.

Child Scenario: You arrive at a residential home as part of an EMS response to a reported electrocution of a 6-year-old child. A BLS engine crew is already performing two-provider CPR. You and your crew are bringing in an AED.

Here are the basic steps to follow during your practice:

PROCEDURE	ACTION
Perform CPR	• Performs ongoing cycles of 30 chest compressions and 2 rescue breaths.
Attach AED	• Turns on AED. • Bares chest. • Adheres pads to chest.
Operate AED	• Stops CPR/movement for analysis. • Clears person and delivers shock. • Immediately begins compressions after shock.
Perform CPR	• Performs ongoing cycles of 30 chest compressions and 2 rescue breaths. • Communicates about switching compressor.
Operate AED / Switch Compressors	• Stops CPR/movement for analysis. • Switches out compressor. • Clears person and delivers shock. • New compressor immediately begins compressions after shock.
Perform CPR	• Performs ongoing cycles of 30 chest compressions and 2 rescue breaths. • Communicates about switching compressor.

The practice will continue without interruption until all of the members of your team, at a minimum, have had the opportunity to play the role of the compressor.

Unique CPR Considerations

Fluids in the Airway

If vomiting has occurred, gurgling is heard, or fluids are visible in the mouth, log roll the person on to his or her side to quickly drain fluids from the mouth. Roll the person without twisting, keeping the head, neck, and torso in line. Remove any material still in the mouth with a gloved finger.

Pregnancy

Chest compressions may not be effective when a woman who is about 20 weeks or more into her pregnancy is lying flat on her back. This is because the fetus puts pressure on a major vein that returns blood to the heart.

Manually displacing the uterus to the mother's left side using one or both hands can move the fetus and relieve the pressure on the vein, improving blood flow from compressions.

Hypothermia

Lower body temperatures can depress body functions and result in clinical signs of respiratory or cardiac arrest. Provide the indicated care and be persistent. Seek active rewarming for the person while continuing care.

If a person is obviously dead, do not start CPR. When defibrillating, if the person does not respond to one shock, focus on continuing CPR and rewarming before repeating the defibrillation.

Electric Shock

Consider any fallen or broken wire extremely dangerous. Do not touch (or allow your clothing to touch) a wire, person, or vehicle that is possibly energized. Do not approach within 8 feet of it. Notify the local utility and have trained personnel sent to scene. NEVER attempt to handle wires yourself unless you are properly trained and equipped.

Electrical shock, even from household current, can result in cardiac or respiratory arrest. As soon as it is safe, assess the person and provide the indicated care. Consider the possibility of spinal injury during care.

Lightning Strike

People struck by lightning are most likely to die from cardiac arrest or persistent respiratory arrest. As soon as it is safe to do so, quickly provide the indicated care. Be persistent. When there are multiple victims, prioritize those in cardiac or respiratory arrest. Consider the possibility of spinal injury during care.

Drowning

Due to the hypoxic nature of drowning, the initial approach focuses on getting rescue breaths initiated as quickly as possible.

With your own safety in mind, remove the person from the water as soon as you can. If trained to do so, and if it does not delay removal, attempt rescue breaths while still in the water.

Do not attempt chest compressions in the water. Do not attempt to remove water from the airway or lungs using abdominal thrusts.

Once a person is removed from the water, immediately assess for normal breathing and pulse. If breathing is absent or only gasping, provide 2 initial rescue breaths that make the chest visibly rise. If the pulse is clearly felt continue with rescue breathing. If a pulse is absent, or if you are not certain, begin CPR. Attach an AED as soon as one is available, drying the chest before applying pads.

Anyone who has received some form of resuscitation for drowning needs to have follow-up evaluation and care in a hospital, regardless of his or her condition after the event.

Injury

Someone in cardiac arrest due to injury is unlikely to survive. If it is clear injury is the cause of arrest, do not start CPR.

Adult BLS Algorithm

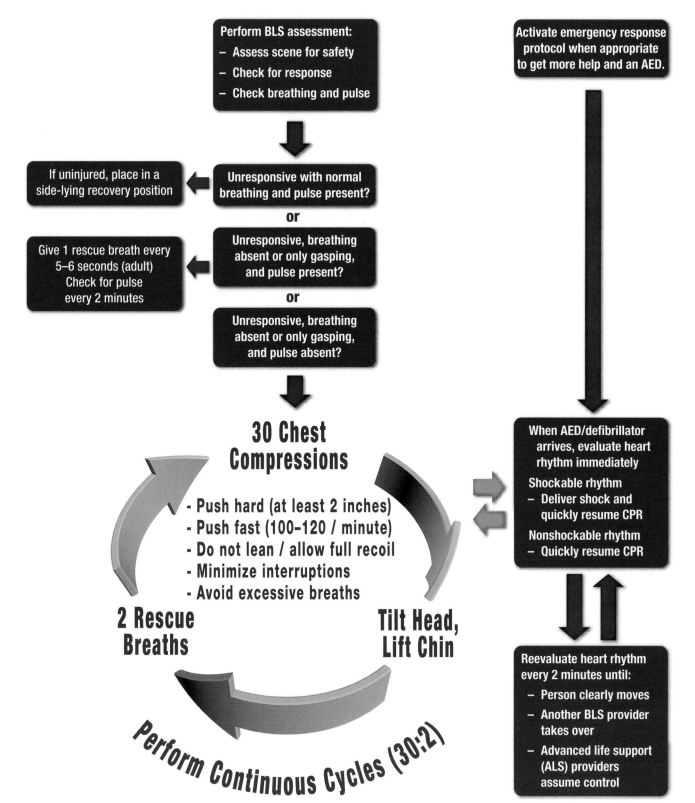

Perform BLS assessment:
- Assess scene for safety
- Check for response
- Check breathing and pulse

Activate emergency response protocol when appropriate to get more help and an AED.

Unresponsive with normal breathing and pulse present?

If uninjured, place in a side-lying recovery position

or

Unresponsive, breathing absent or only gasping, and pulse present?

Give 1 rescue breath every 5–6 seconds (adult) Check for pulse every 2 minutes

or

Unresponsive, breathing absent or only gasping, and pulse absent?

30 Chest Compressions

- Push hard (at least 2 inches)
- Push fast (100–120 / minute)
- Do not lean / allow full recoil
- Minimize interruptions
- Avoid excessive breaths

2 Rescue Breaths

Tilt Head, Lift Chin

Perform Continuous Cycles (30:2)

When AED/defibrillator arrives, evaluate heart rhythm immediately

Shockable rhythm
- Deliver shock and quickly resume CPR

Nonshockable rhythm
- Quickly resume CPR

Reevaluate heart rhythm every 2 minutes until:
- Person clearly moves
- Another BLS provider takes over
- Advanced life support (ALS) providers assume control

BLS Summary

	ADULT	CHILD	INFANT
Age Determination	Begins with onset of puberty	About 1 year of age to the onset of puberty	Less than 1 year of age
Scene Safety?	If the scene is unsafe or at anytime becomes unsafe, GET OUT!	If the scene is unsafe or at anytime becomes unsafe, GET OUT!	If the scene is unsafe or at anytime becomes unsafe, GET OUT!
Response?	Tap shoulder, shout name	Tap shoulder, shout name	Tap foot, shout out
Breathing and Pulse?	• Look at face and chest for no breathing or only gasping • Palpate for carotid pulse • Take no more than 10 seconds to check	• Look at face and chest for no breathing or only gasping • Palpate for carotid pulse • Take no more than 10 seconds to check	• Look at face and chest for no breathing or only gasping • Palpate for brachial pulse • Take no more than 10 seconds to check
Activate Emergency Response Protocol and get an AED	Accomplish given the circumstances and protocols of your situation	Accomplish given the circumstances and protocols of your situation	Accomplish given the circumstances and protocols of your situation
Normal Breathing Present! Pulse Present!	Place person in recovery position and monitor breathing	Place child in recovery position and monitor breathing	Place infant in recovery position and monitor breathing
Normal Breathing Absent! Pulse Present!	• Perform rescue breathing; 1 breath every 5–6 seconds • Monitor carotid pulse every 2 minutes	• If pulse is 60 beats per minute or greater, perform rescue breathing; 1 breath every 3–5 seconds • Monitor carotid pulse every 2 minutes	• If pulse is 60 beats per minute or greater, perform rescue breathing; 1 breath every 3–5 seconds • Monitor brachial pulse every 2 minutes
Rescue Breaths	• Tilt head, lift chin to open airway first • 1 second in length • Make chest visibly rise, but no more	• Tilt head, lift chin to open airway first • 1 second in length • Make chest visibly rise, but no more	• Tilt head, lift chin to open airway first • 1 second in length • Make chest visibly rise, but no more
Normal Breathing Absent! Pulse Absent!	• Perform CPR starting with compressions • Single or multiple providers — provide continuous cycles of 30 compressions and 2 rescue breaths	• If pulse is absent, or less than 60 BPM with poor perfusion, perform CPR starting with compressions • Single provider — provide continuous cycles of 30:2 • Multiple providers — provide continuous cycles of 15:2	• If pulse is absent, or less than 60 BPM with poor perfusion, perform CPR starting with compressions • Single provider — provide continuous cycles of 30:2 • Multiple providers — provide continuous cycles of 15:2
Compressions	• 2 hands on center of chest, lower half of breastbone • At least 2 inches in depth • Rate of 100–120 times per minute • Deep, fast, full rebound, minimize interruption	• 1 or 2 hands on lower half of breastbone • At least $\frac{1}{3}$ diameter of chest or about 2 inches in depth • Rate of 100–120 times per minute • Deep, fast, full rebound, minimize interruption	• 2 fingers on breastbone just below nipple line • At least 1/3 diameter of chest or about 1 1/2 inches in depth • Rate of 100–120 times per minute • Deep, fast, full rebound, minimize interruption
Defibrillation with AED	• Turn on power • Attach pads • Analyze • If indicated, deliver shock • Immediately resume CPR • Follow voice instructions	• Use pediatric system; if not available, use AED for adult • Turn on power • Attach pads • Analyze • If indicated, deliver shock • Immediately resume CPR • Follow voice instructions	• Use pediatric system; if not available, use AED for adult • Turn on power • Attach pads • Analyze • If indicated, deliver shock • Immediately resume CPR • Follow voice instructions

Choking

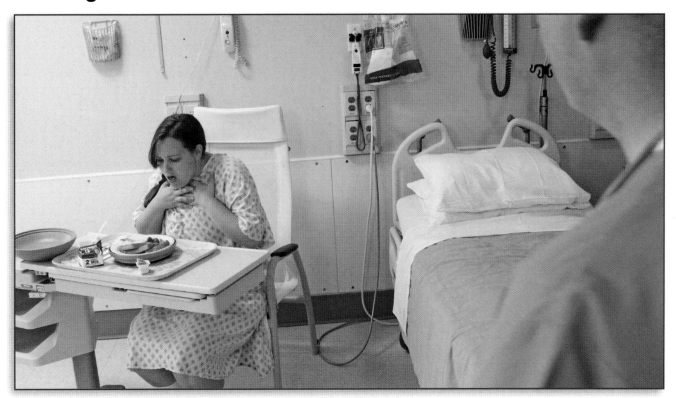

Choking can occur when a solid object, such as a piece of food or a small object, enters a narrowed part of the airway and becomes stuck. On inhalation, the object can be drawn tighter into the airway and block air from entering the lungs.

A forceful thrust beneath the ribs and up into the diaphragm can pressurize the air in the chest and pop an obstruction out of the airway. Compression of the chest over the breastbone can also create enough pressure to expel an object.

Mild Obstruction

To provide the appropriate care, you must first be able to recognize the difference between a mild blockage and a severe blockage.

With a mild blockage, a person can speak, cough, or gag. This type of obstruction is typically cleared by the affected person naturally through forceful coughing. Allow someone with a mild blockage to try and resolve the problem on his or her own. Stay close and be ready to take action if things worsen.

Severe Obstruction

When a severe blockage occurs, a person cannot take in enough air to dislodge the object. Signs of severe obstruction include very little or no air exchange, the lack of sound, and the inability to speak or cough forcefully. The person may hold his or her hands to the throat while attempting to clear the obstruction.

A person without any air exchange requires your help to survive. Repeated abdominal thrusts, given by standing behind someone and wrapping your arms around him or her, have shown to be extremely effective in relieving a severe foreign-body airway obstruction.

Blind Finger Sweeps

It is not recommended to use blind finger sweeps to check for foreign objects in the airway.

When someone is clearly pregnant or obese, use chest thrusts instead of abdominal thrusts. Position yourself directly behind the person. Reach under the armpits and place the thumb side of your fist on the center of the chest. Grasp your fist with your other hand and thrust straight backward. Try to not put pressure on the ribs.

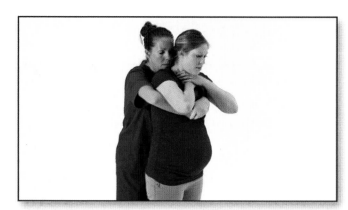

If you are choking and alone, try pressing your abdomen quickly against a rigid surface, such as falling on to the back of a chair. If one is not available, attempt abdominal thrusts on yourself.

Abdominal and chest thrusts can cause internal injury. Anyone who has had these maneuvers used on them should be evaluated further to ensure there are no injuries.

Children and Infants

Young children are particularly at risk for choking because of the small size of their air passages, inexperience with chewing, and a natural tendency to put objects in their mouths.

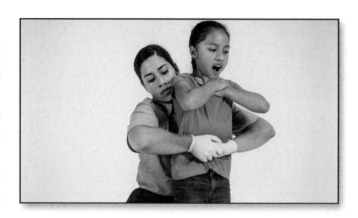

For a choking child, the approach is nearly the same as for adults. It might be easier to kneel behind a choking child to deliver thrusts. Use less force on your thrusts.

Because infants do not speak, it may be more difficult to recognize choking. A sudden onset differentiates it from other breathing emergencies. Signs include weak, ineffective coughs, and the lack of sound, even when an infant is clearly attempting to breathe.

If Alone

If you are alone with someone who collapses during your choking treatment, perform 2 minutes of CPR before you activate your emergency response protocol and get an AED yourself.

Knowledge Check

You are in the hospital cafeteria eating lunch with a coworker. He is laughing at something you said when he suddenly stops, grasps his throat with his hands, and stands up quickly. He clearly looks distressed so you stand up next to him and ask, "Are you choking?" He nods yes to you and is completely silent. Describe how to care for him.

ADDITIONAL CONSIDERATIONS

Choking — Adults and Children

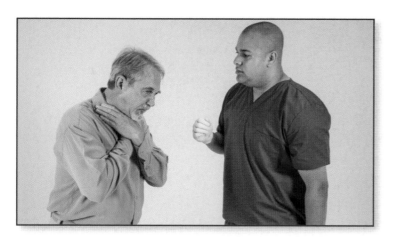

Assess Person

- Ask, "Are you choking?"
- If person nods yes, or is unable to speak or cough, act quickly.
- If available, have someone activate your emergency response protocol.

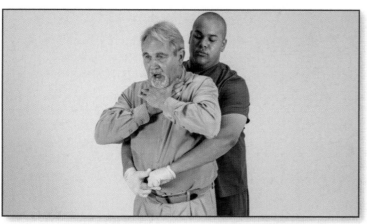

Position Yourself

- Stand behind person. If needed, kneel behind a child.
- Reach around and locate navel.
- Make a fist with other hand and place thumb side against abdomen, just above navel and below ribs.
- Grasp fist with other hand.

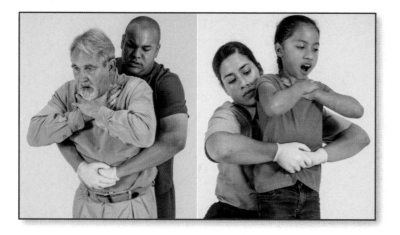

Give Thrusts

- Quickly thrust inward and upward into abdomen.
- Repeat. Each thrust needs to be given with intent of expelling object.
- Continue until person can breathe normally.

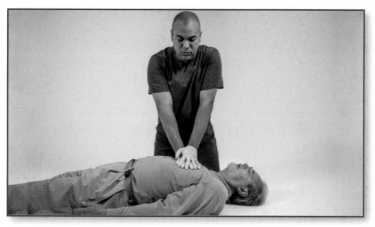

If Person Becomes Unresponsive

- Carefully lower person to ground.
- Begin CPR, starting with compressions.
- Look in mouth for an object before giving rescue breaths. Remove any object seen.
- Continue until another BLS provider takes over, the person shows signs of life, or you are too exhausted to continue.

Choking — Infants

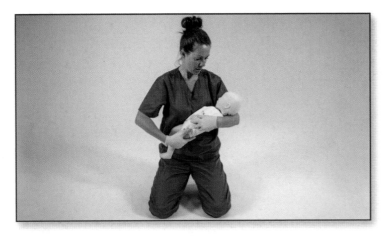

Assess Infant

- Look at infant's face.
- If infant has weak, ineffective coughs, or lack of sound even when clearly attempting to breathe, act quickly!
- If available, have someone activate your emergency response protocol.

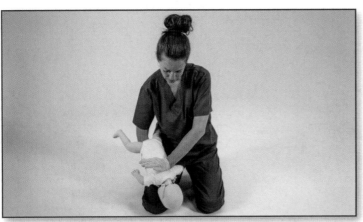

Give 5 Back Blows

- Lay infant face down over your forearm with legs straddled and with head lower than the chest. Support the head by holding the jaw.
- Using heel of other hand, give 5 back blows between shoulder blades.

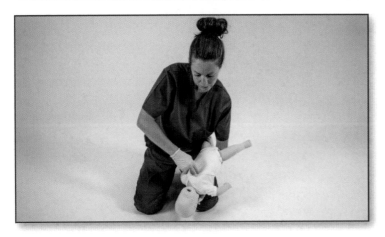

Give 5 Chest Thrusts

- Sandwich infant between your forearms and turn onto back.
- Place 2 fingertips on breastbone just below nipple line and give 5 chest thrusts.
- Repeat back blows and chest thrusts until infant can breathe normally.

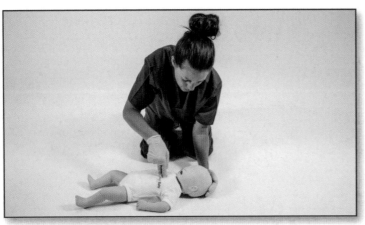

If Infant Becomes Unresponsive

- Gently place infant on firm surface.
- Look in mouth for an object before giving rescue breaths. Remove any object seen.
- Continue until another BLS provider takes over, the person shows signs of life, or you are too exhausted to continue.

Legal Considerations

Good Samaritan Laws

All states have passed what are known as Good Samaritan laws to encourage bystanders and off-duty BLS providers to assist those in need. These laws help protect anyone who

- voluntarily provides assistance, without expecting or accepting compensation,
- is reasonable and prudent,
- does not provide care beyond the training received, and
- is not grossly negligent, or completely careless, in delivering emergency care.

Good Samaritan laws vary slightly from state to state. Become familiar with the laws in your state and other states where you work or travel.

Abandonment

Once care has begun, and it is safe to do so, remain with the person until someone with equal or greater emergency medical training takes over. If alone, it is okay to leave to activate EMS, but return to the person as soon as you can.

Consent

It is appropriate to ask a responsive person if they want help before providing care. To get consent, first identify yourself. Then tell the person your level of training and ask if it's okay to help. Implied consent means that permission to provide care to an unresponsive person is assumed. This is based on the idea that a reasonable person would give permission to receive lifesaving care if able. Consent for children must be gained from a parent or legal guardian. When life-threatening situations exist and the parent or guardian is not available, care should be given based on implied consent. When suffering from a disturbance in normal mental functioning, like Alzheimer's disease, a person may not understand your request for consent. Consent must be gained from a family member or legal guardian.

Duty to Act

This is a requirement to act toward others and the public with the watchfulness, attention, caution and prudence that a reasonable person in the same circumstances would use. If a person's actions do not meet this standard, then the acts may be considered negligent, and any damages resulting may be claimed in a lawsuit for negligence. If you are a state licensed healthcare provider, first responder, or other professional rescuer expected to give emergency medical care, including CPR, you almost certainly have a duty to act. However, BLS performed voluntarily on a stranger in need while off duty is generally considered a Good Samaritan act.

Assault and Battery

A criminal act of placing a person in fear of bodily harm. A conscious and aware adult has the right to refuse medical treatment. Forcing care on a person against his or her wishes may be considered grounds for this.

Starting CPR

Start CPR for anyone in cardiac arrest unless obvious signs of death are present, including rigor mortis (limbs of corpse stiff and are impossible to move), dependent lividity (settling of blood in lower portions of body causing a purplish red discoloration), or when conditions are present that are incompatible with life (decomposition, decapitation, massive head injury, etc.). Do not start CPR if it puts you in danger of injury, or the person has a valid do not resuscitate (DNR) order. In a mass casualty incident with limited resources, people requiring rescue breathing or CPR are considered dead and attempts to resuscitate them should not be started.

Stopping CPR

Do not stop CPR until a healthcare provider or other professional rescuer with equal or more training takes over, you are exhausted, the scene becomes too dangerous to continue, or the person being treated shows signs of life. You can also stop if directed to do so by the physician in charge of patient care for the person. Except when death is obvious, irreversible brain damage or brain death cannot be reliably assessed or predicted. Providers should never make an impulsive decision about the present or future quality of life for a person in cardiac arrest because such decisions may be incorrect.

Advanced Directives and Living Wills

These are documents authorized by state law that allow a person to appoint someone as his or her representative to make decisions on resuscitation and continued life support in a situation where a person has lost decision-making capacity (for example, if unresponsive). These documents may also be referred to as a durable power of attorney. Advanced directives are statements about what a person wants done or not done when he or she can't speak on his or her own behalf. Laws about advanced directives are different in each state. You should be aware of the laws in your state.

Do Not Resuscitate (DNR) or Do Not Attempt Resuscitation (DNAR) Orders

The DNR/DNAR order is a kind of advanced directive. This is a specific request not to have CPR performed. In the United States, a doctor's order is required to withhold CPR. Therefore, unless the person has a DNR order, EMS providers and hospital staff should attempt resuscitation. People who are not likely to benefit from CPR and may have a DNR include those with terminal conditions. Outside the hospital, healthcare providers, first responders, and other professional rescuers should begin CPR if there is a reasonable doubt about the validity of a DNR or advanced directive, if the person may have changed his or her mind, or the person's best interests are in question.

ADDITIONAL CONSIDERATIONS

Glossary

abdominal thrust

Thrusts administered to the abdomen of a responsive, choking person to dislodge an object blocking a person's airway.

acute coronary syndrome (ACS)

Often described as a heart attack, ACS occurs when there is reduced blood flow to the tissues of the heart.

advanced airway

A device placed into the trachea or esophagus to allow direct ventilation into the lungs while helping to prevent aspiration of fluids or foreign material.

agonal breaths

Weak, irregular gasping, snorting, or gurgling sounds that can occur early in cardiac arrest. They provide no usable oxygen and are not normal breathing.

airway

The passageway between mouth and lungs that allows life-sustaining oxygen into the body.

automated external defibrillator (AED)

A small, portable, computerized device that allows a minimally trained bystander to provide defibrillation much faster than EMS.

AED operator

Provider tasked with the efficient and safe delivery of AED defibrillation shocks in a team approach to resuscitation.

bag mask

Rescue breathing device with a pliable, refilling bag that can be squeezed to force air out through a connected mask.

bloodborne pathogens

Infectious microorganisms in human blood that can cause disease in humans. These pathogens include hepatitis B (HBV), hepatitis C (HCV) and human immunodeficiency virus (HIV).

BLS assessment

An assessment to quickly identify if a basic life support is present.

brachial pulse

Heartbeat pulsations of the brachial arteries that can be felt on both inner, upper arms.

cardiopulmonary resuscitation (CPR)

A combination of rescue breaths and chest compressions performed on a person experiencing cardiac arrest, intended to restore some oxygen to the brain.

carotid pulse

Heartbeat pulsations of the carotid arteries that can be felt on both sides of the neck between the muscles on the sides of the neck and the trachea in the front.

chain of survival

A concept of 5 interdependent links that describe the most effective approach for treating sudden cardiac arrest. Versions include outside the hospital for adults, inside the hospital for adults, and one for children and infants.

chest compression

A basic CPR skill that creates increased pressure in the chest cavity and direct compression of the heart. This forces blood to move from the chest to the lungs, brain, and rest of the body.

chest thrust

Thrusts administered on the breastbone of a responsive, choking person to dislodge an object stuck in the person's airway.

compression-only CPR

A simple, but limited, approach to treating sudden cardiac arrest that is being widely promoted to people who are not formally trained in CPR.

compressor

Provider tasked with performing chest compressions while another provider gives rescue breaths during two-provider CPR.

CPR feedback device

Device that can measure skill performance during CPR such as depth, rate, timing, and recoil.

CPR mask

A protective barrier device used to prevent exposure to potentially infectious body fluids while performing rescue breaths on a person. The mask fits over the mouth and nose of the person and includes a one-way valve to blow through.

defibrillation

The delivery of an electrical shock through the heart intended to end chaotic electrical activity in the heart and allow the heart's normal electrical activity to return.

emergency medical services (EMS)

An emergency medical response system developed within a community, consisting of a specialized communications network and trained professional responders, all accessible through an emergency phone number such as 911.

emergency response protocols

Predetermined guidelines on how to alert other providers and get additional resuscitation equipment, such as an AED, in an emergency.

femoral pulse

Heartbeat pulsations of the femoral arteries that can be felt just below the middle of the crease where the leg and torso meet.

Good Samaritan law

A law enacted to legally protect trained providers who voluntarily stop to help, act prudently, do not provide care beyond training, and are not completely careless in delivering emergency care.

head tilt-chin lift

The recommended technique to open and maintain the airway of an unresponsive person. It pulls the jaw forward and lifts the tongue away from the back of the throat.

heart attack

See acute coronary syndrome.

high-performance CPR (HPCPR)

A combination of high-quality CPR skills and an integrated team approach to resuscitation intended to improve a person's chance of surviving cardiac arrest.

implied consent

A legal concept referring to the assumption that an unresponsive person would give permission to be helped if responsive.

jaw thrust

A technique to open the airway with a provider located above the person's head, using a CPR mask or bag mask to deliver rescue breaths. The head is tilted and the jaw is thrust upwards using fingertips on the bottom of the jaw, just below the ear.

jaw thrust without head tilt

The jaw thrust airway technique without tilting the head back. Used when an injury to the neck is suspected.

naloxone

A medication that can temporarily reverse the life-threatening effects of opioids. It is administered either through an auto-injector device or through an aerosol that is sprayed into the nose. Naloxone is becoming more readily available to lay providers.

opioid

Pain medication that can depress and even stop breathing when taken in overdose.

protective barrier

An item that helps reduce the risk of exposure to blood and other potentially infectious body fluids. Examples include disposable gloves, CPR masks, and face shields.

recovery position

A side-lying position in which an unresponsive breathing person is placed to drain fluids from the mouth and keep the tongue from blocking the airway.

rescue breathing

Indicated treatment for respiratory arrest in which ongoing rescue breaths are provided.

rescue breaths

Artificial breaths given to someone who is not breathing, administered by blowing air into the mouth to inflate the lungs.

respiratory arrest

A life-threatening BLS emergency in which breathing is absent or not normal and the heart is still beating.

secondary cardiac arrest

The loss of measurable signs of life as the end result of a blocked airway or loss of breathing.

standard precautions

A consistent set of protective practices used whether or not an infection is suspected. The approach is the same for everyone, regardless of relationship or age.

sudden cardiac arrest (SCA)

The abrupt loss of the heart's ability to contract and push blood forward through the circulatory system. Typically caused by a sudden disruption of the heart's electrical system.

team leader

Provider tasked with taking a general perspective to supervise and improve overall performance in a team approach to resuscitation.

unresponsive

A condition in which a person does not respond to physical or verbal attempts to get a response.

ventilator

Provider tasked with giving rescue breaths while another provider performs chest compressions during two-provider CPR.

ventricular fibrillation

A chaotic, quivering heart rhythm that prevents the normal contraction of the heart and the ability to pump blood.

Sources

The Basic Life Support Student Book is based upon the following standards, guidelines, and recommendations:

2015 International Consensus on Cardiopulmonary Resuscitation and Emergency Cardiovascular Care Science With Treatment Recommendations. Circulation 132, suppl 1 (2015):S2–S268.

2015 International Consensus on First Aid Science With Treatment Recommendations. Circulation 132, suppl 1 (2015):S269–S311.

2015 American Heart Association Guidelines Update for Cardiopulmonary Resuscitation and Emergency Cardiovascular Care. Circulation 132, suppl 2 (2015):S315–S573.

2015 American Heart Association and American Red Cross Guidelines Update for First Aid. Circulation 132, suppl 2 (2015): S574–S589.

ANSI/ASSE. Z490.1-2016: Criteria for Accepted Practices in Safety, Health, & Environmental Training Standard. Park Ridge, IL: ASSE, 2016.

ASTM International. F2171-02 Standard Guide for Defining the Performance of First Aid Providers in Occupational Settings. West Conshohocken, PA: ASTM International, 2009.

U.S. Occupational Safety and Health Administration. Best Practices Guide: Fundamentals of a Workplace First-Aid Program. OSHA 3317-06N. Washington DC: Department of Labor, 2006.

Endnotes

1. "Latex Allergy," MedlinePlus Medical Encyclopedia, U.S. National Library of Medicine, last updated March 9, 2016, https://www.nlm.nih.gov/medlineplus/latexallergy.html.

ADDITIONAL INFORMATION

Knowledge Check Answers

Sudden Cardiac Arrest — *Page 2*

Defibrillation. A controlled electrical shock is sent through the heart to stop ventricular fibrillation, allowing the heart's normal electrical activity to return and restore the normal pumping action of the heart.

Secondary Cardiac Arrest — *Page 4*

Drowning is a common cause of secondary cardiac arrest in which the heart becomes progressively weaker from the lack of oxygen. Immediate CPR with an emphasis on high-quality rescue breaths may provide his only chance for survival.

High-Performance CPR — *Page 6*

High-quality CPR skills and an integrated team approach much like a pit crew in a car race.

Protecting Yourself — *Page 8*

False. Standard precautions is a set of protective practices used whether or not an infection is suspected. To be effective, your approach is the same for everyone, regardless of situation or age.

Calling for Help — *Page 9*

An EMS provider may request help from more advanced EMS providers or inform other incoming BLS responders about the details of the situation found.

Chest Compressions — *Page 11*

1. Compress deeply, more than 2 inches.
2. Compress fast, between 100 and 120 times per minute.
3. Do not lean on the chest between compressions.
4. Minimize interruptions while doing compressions.

Rescue Breaths — *Page 15*

Each breath should be about 1 second in length, and only have enough air to create a visible rise of the chest, but no more. Additional air is unnecessary.

Automated External Defibrillation — *Page 21*

1. Turn on the AED.
2. Adhere defibrillation pads to his bare chest.
3. Allow the AED to analyze his heart rhythm.
4. Deliver a shock if directed to by the AED.

BLS Assessment — *Page 25*

Perform CPR immediately, starting with compressions. Irregular gasping, snorting, or gurgling sounds do not provide oxygen and do not indicate normal breathing.

Caring for Respiratory Arrest — *Page 28*

You will provide a single rescue breath every 5 to 6 seconds, or about 10 to 12 breaths per minute. You will also monitor the pulse about every 2 minutes.

Caring for Cardiac Arrest — *Page 32*

Begin CPR starting with compressions. Perform ongoing cycles of 30 chest compressions and 2 rescue breaths. Stop CPR when the AED is attached and ready to analyze. Deliver a defibrillation shock if directed to by the AED.

Multiple Provider Approach to CPR — *Page 38*

True. When 2 more providers are available to perform CPR, compressions and breaths should be split between the providers.

Choking — *Page 46*

Stand behind him. Reach around and locate his navel with your finger. Make a fist with your other hand and place the thumb side against the abdomen, just above your finger and below his ribs. Grasp your fist with the other hand and give a quick inward and upward thrust to expel the obstruction. Repeat thrusts until he can breathe normally.

Rate Your Program

This course evaluation allows you to rate the training course you have just completed. This evaluation will provide your training provider with feedback on the quality of the instruction you received.

Program Name _____ □ ASHI □ MEDIC First Aid

Instructor _____ Date of Course_____

Please rate the following course elements as indicated below. Place a check in the box that best represents your opinion of the quality of each element. *Thank you for your help.*	4–Excellent	3–Good	2–Average	1–Poor
Course Presentation				
Organization, pace, and flow	□	□	□	□
Not too basic, not too complex	□	□	□	□
Time allowed for skill practice	□	□	□	□
Increased your confidence and ability to take action	□	□	□	□
Instructor(s)				
Subject knowledge	□	□	□	□
Teaching ability (clear, concise, organized)	□	□	□	□
Demeanor (friendly, helpful, engaging)	□	□	□	□
Program Materials				
Video	□	□	□	□
PowerPoint®	□	□	□	□
Student Book	□	□	□	□
Online Training Component (if taken)	□	□	□	□
Location and Equipment				
Space	□	□	□	□
Training equipment	□	□	□	□
Self Assessment				
How would you rate your emergency care skills BEFORE taking this class?	□	□	□	□
How would you rate your emergency care skills AFTER taking this class?	□	□	□	□
How willing would you be to respond in an emergency BEFORE taking this class?	□	□	□	□
How willing would you be to respond in an emergency AFTER taking this class?	□	□	□	□
Your overall score for the course	□	□	□	□

What did you like most about this course? _____

_____

What did you like least about this course? _____

_____

Would you recommend this course to others?   □ Yes   □ No

Student input is an essential aspect of our ongoing quality assurance efforts. HSI requires that students be given the opportunity to evaluate their ASHI or MEDIC First Aid course using this Rate Your Program course evaluation form. You may also provide feedback directly to HSI at www.hsi.com/rateyourprogram.